Aromatherapy and Women's Mental Health

AROMATHERAPY and WOMEN'S MENTAL HEALTH

An Evidence-Based Guide to Support Emotional Wellbeing

PAM CONRAD

Foreword by Denise Tiran
Illustrations by Courtney Merino

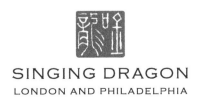

SINGING DRAGON
LONDON AND PHILADELPHIA

First published in Great Britain in 2023 by Singing Dragon,
an imprint of Jessica Kingsley Publishers
Part of John Murray Press

1

A CIP catalogue record for this title is available from the
British Library and the Library of Congress

ISBN 978 1 83997 624 7
eISBN 978 1 83997 625 4

Printed and bound in the United States by Integrated Books International

Jessica Kingsley Publishers' policy is to use papers that are natural,
renewable and recyclable products and made from wood grown in
sustainable forests. The logging and manufacturing processes are expected
to conform to the environmental regulations of the country of origin.

Singing Dragon
Carmelite House
50 Victoria Embankment
London EC4Y 0DZ

www.singingdragon.com

John Murray Press
Part of Hodder & Stoughton Limited
An Hachette UK Company

Dedicated to the stars of my life, Katie and Ryan,
who enrich my heart and bring me great joy!

Contents

Foreword

I am delighted to have been asked to contribute the foreword to Pam's latest book. I first met Pam in 2002, when she contacted me while studying a degree in complementary therapies in London, UK. Pam asked to observe my complementary therapy midwifery teaching clinic for expectant mothers, which was part of my work at the University of Greenwich, London. Pam joined me in the clinic every Monday for almost a year – and a firm friendship was formed, as well as a mutual professional respect. Having known her now for over 20 years, I know that Pam is a sensitive and caring person who is totally committed to holistic care. While mental health is the "hot topic" for the current decade, Pam has always been dedicated to ensuring that women's healthcare involves not only the physiological aspects, but also the psychological and spiritual elements. She demonstrates this on a daily basis, in her clinical practice, her teaching and her publications, as well as in her faith.

Aromatherapy and Women's Mental Health is a very readable text and Pam gives of herself in this immensely personal book. For her readers, she skilfully and seamlessly weaves together the two healthcare disciplines of women's health and aromatherapy.

Indeed, it is this application of the one to the other that is so essential to professional learning, helping nurses and midwives to appreciate fully the benefits of using essential oils and massage across the wide spectrum from menarche to menopause and beyond. The inclusion of physiopathology and psychology, as well as chemical aromatherapy research, lifts this book to the professional level required by nurses, while retaining its reader-friendly approach, making it suitable also for women who may want to self-administer essential oils. I particularly like the inclusion of the case studies to illustrate the effectiveness of aromatherapy for a variety of mental health issues, and the progression through the female life cycle, including motherhood and the use of essential oils in children and teenagers.

Dr Denise Tiran, HonDUniv, FRCM, MSc, RM, PGCEA,
London, UK, 2023
CEO/Education Director, Expectancy
www.expectancy.co.uk
International lecturer in midwifery complementary therapies
info@expectancy.co.uk

Introduction

Let's shine a light on mental health and the therapeutic space aromatherapy can fill

As I begin this book, the world is slowly emerging from a two-year pandemic, facing a brutal war and unprecedented rates of mental health issues. We've experienced considerable personal and collective loss with tolls on our physical and emotional health and overall wellbeing. Recent data indicates children and teens' rates of suicide attempts have increased by 50 percent with emergency room records indicating daily suicide attempts related to significant decreased social interaction, unnatural isolation with remote education and social media often the only means of peer communication (Department of Health and Human Services/Centers for Disease Control and Prevention 2021). A sense of urgency drives me to write this guidebook, to share years of nursing experience supporting mental health along with 20 years of successful clinical nursing aromatherapy experiences. My goal is to reach those needing support to ease anxiety, depression, fears, panic, loss and grief on its own or alongside any number of medical conditions and life circumstances. Aromatherapy, as will be shared in this guidebook, is effective, safe, affordable, accessible and, as a bonus, smells nice and enhances our personal and professional environments. The published studies, *the evidence base*, will highlight and affirm the decades of positive responses from thousands of patients and clients receiving aromatherapy treatments, and the practical, published and anecdotal will be shared in equal measure.

My personal experience

At the age of five, I had my first brush with mental health, or lack thereof, with a family secret, a dark misunderstood secret: "What really happened to Grandpa?" A Midwest farmer, my maternal grandfather died from suicide, and no one would speak of it for decades, though it was impossible not to feel the shift in our family. Somewhere deep inside me, the seeds were planted that bad things can happen if you don't take care of your thoughts and feelings—your emotional health—just like you do your physical health, unnecessary and painful losses can occur, changing the fiber of a family forever.

My childhood was spent in our family pharmacy listening alongside my father to the myriad of people's physical discomforts and requests for medications and remedies to smooth the rough patches. The human condition and accompanying people through their journey always appealed to me, both in the pharmacy and at our kitchen table, with the neighbor ladies sharing their confidences and occasional family secrets. In a culture of shame and secrecy about any mental health issues, the private world of women's trusted relationships around quilting circles, coffee shops, book clubs and glasses of wine was and is a true and valuable form of therapy, a saving grace for countless women in times of crisis.

In those years, the desire to help people feel better by listening, sharing, keeping confidences or making a concoction continued to flourish as I chose my career path in healthcare. Weaving together pharmacy and kitchen-table confidences from childhood, nursing and aromatherapy provided me with ideal modalities for women's and family mental health care.

As a nursing student at Purdue, I was particularly drawn to and a bit afraid of psychiatric nursing. In the 1980s we still had large state hospitals with evidence of past lobotomy and shock ECT treatment areas. My beautiful, kind great aunt, sister of my grandfather, jumped to her death in a well on her farm after decades of grief from the tragic losses of her two young children and ensuing shock treatments. She swore she'd never endure those treatments again and at that time the only other options were psychiatric medications or institutions. She maintained her physical beauty and warm, joyful spirit, expertly hiding her unrelenting sadness until she could no longer survive the pain. Her physical beauty and charming personality impressed upon me as a young woman that even those who appear to have it all together can still be deeply suffering. This event cemented in me the importance of lifelong emotional self-care and to be an advocate for mental health. I encourage strangers, friends and family to get help when needed, go to therapy, communicate openly, search for remedies, food, supplementation, exercise and activities that enhance joy! Having people you can trust in your life whenever you need them is invaluable.

Mental health treatments have progressed and are more

humane, although they continue to carry a stigma, with serious risks that this creates an inability to access much needed support and treatment. This reality is the reason I'm writing this book to open dialogue, and offer resources, options and complementary therapies, particularly aromatherapy, for self-care. Clinically, mental health is not solely in one locked unit of a hospital or facility on the outskirts of town; it exists in every unit with every condition as well as in our homes, schools, churches and communities. Outcomes in all scenarios and conditions are improved if emotional harmony is the goal. Our mental health needs daily care just like our physical health and needs to be taught alongside basic care and hygiene. A mild headache is not acute pain, but we pay attention to it, alter our food, supplement, increase our fluid intake, grab a Tylenol, rest and access professional help when needed. Asking others, "Is everything ok?" "How are you doing?" "I'm here if you need to talk," "Did something happen today?" and sharing "Some days can be particularly tough," "How can I help?" and by the end of this book, "Would you like to smell something nice?" are all needed in daily life.

The focus is on women's mental health and aromatherapy; however, women are mothers to both males and females, wives, sisters, daughters, girlfriends: they care for everyone in their realm. Other than the specific studies on women's reproductive health conditions, virtually all of the oils and methodology of treatments in this book are effective, appropriate and recommended for everyone. Professionals seeking information on treatments for both males and females can comfortably follow the shared aromatherapy evidence base and practice tips for anxiety and depression for both genders.

The human condition includes a vast array of emotions, just as Mother Nature's garden includes bark, leaves, needles, sap, flowers, leaves, seeds, cones, roots and berries full of intricate components for the plants' survival as well as therapeutic value for humans. The pleasurable sensations one feels from the scents wafting through the forest on a nature hike, a rose bouquet from a lover or cinnamon rolls baking in the oven highlight the provocative effect of our sense of smell. These emotions can be invoked with essential oils from these plants, triggering positive memories, uplifting spirits and tapping into long-ago mind–body sensations. The therapeutic value of aromatherapy is particularly beneficial with mental and emotional health and this guidebook will demonstrate this from the evidence base as well as case studies and tips from years of practice.

Aromatherapy is not a cure or replacement for medical or psychological evaluation and treatment. All serious mental health conditions, those dark scary places one's mind can take an individual, or any inability caused by emotions to function normally for two consecutive weeks, needs a professional evaluation. Crisis centers are a phone call away and anytime a person considers self-harm or harming others, a crisis call and follow-up professional evaluation are the most important actions for everyone! Having said this, the wait for many people needing attention is too long, so a toolkit of self-care therapies offers support to decrease anxiety and panic and uplift depression even if this is simply until they can get additional care. In visions of a more humane world, there could be lavender or citrus "sniff stations" in bathrooms, schools and workplaces.

Let's start from the very beginning…in the perfect future world, a newly pregnant woman would be asked about her emotional health, complete brief standardized anxiety and depression questionnaires and review her history. She would be educated about the shifting hormonal changes of pregnancy that can and often do affect emotions, and how fears and anxiety along with excitement are all normal. Caring for the woman's emotions from her first appointment through a year postpartum to provide her and her family with the best possible start and education on the importance and value of her lifelong emotional health will carry over to her family members' mental health. From the beginning of life, pediatricians will discuss emotions, behavioral changes at various ages, importance of communication and coping mechanisms. At home, in schools, activity clubs, teams and churches there will be communication about life events, relationships, losses, disappointments and how all can affect feelings.

My professional experience

As a senior nursing student, I was the only one in the class to raise my hand for what my professor referred to as an "amazing opportunity" to spend an entire semester in a psychiatrist practice, learning individual and group therapy as well as accompanying him on hospital patient rounds. At the time and until very recently, mental health centers existed on the fringes of medicine, with separate facilities tucked away on manicured hillsides on the outskirts of town. Although quite an upgrade from the soon-to-close state hospitals, the messaging was still clear that these people needed to be outside of society, outside of medicine.

A brilliant psychiatrist, albeit a sadly broken man with a tragic backstory, he taught me a great deal that semester.

However, due to my youth and lack of life experiences, I chose not to enter the mental health field at that point. As a graduate nurse, at the tender age of 21, I feared I would be swallowed up by the "darkness" of it all, and the regular reassurances of "You're such a natural at this" were far from comforting. Aside from the therapy skills I acquired, the most valuable lesson I've carried forward to this day was that all people have a story—behind their behaviors, expressed symptoms and diagnosis, there's a back story to most aspects of their lives.

After four years in emergency trauma and cardiology nursing, I practiced inpatient psychiatric nursing for several years and thereafter have woven mental health into every aspect of my career. With group therapy skills, I co-facilitated cancer and women's health support groups, and individual therapy skills accompanied me daily in conventional medical as well as complementary therapy consultations. In 2000, I completed an 18-month clinical aromatherapy for healthcare professionals program, which beautifully weaves the physical, emotional and spiritual realms of the human condition together. With the additional tools of clinical aromatherapy in my years of individual consultations, group therapy sessions, and direct patient care, I've witnessed rapid decreases in anxiety, fear and panic, uplifting of depressive symptoms, and improved physical conditions. Overall, enhanced communication about difficult, deeply hidden, painful and often unspoken topics have paved a way to healing. Aromatherapy, particularly by inhalation, simply "peels the onion" much more quickly and as a therapist, preparation and respect for these actions is a worthy tip for practice!

In 2001, after becoming certified in clinical aromatherapy, I studied advanced aromatherapy and graduate complementary therapy studies in England for two years. Since the late 1980s, midwives and nurses educated in maternity and oncology aromatherapy had developed well-established clinical programs throughout the country, published large clinical aromatherapy research studies, and were my mentors as I began my women's health nursing aromatherapy practice. In 2004, returning to the US, based on their decades of evidence-based practice and successful program development, I developed an evidence-based nursing aromatherapy curriculum endorsed by the American Holistic Nurses Association (AHNA) and American College of Nurse Midwives (ACNM) and educated multiple nurses and midwives to develop hospital nursing aromatherapy and pharmacy programs in hospice, obstetrics and outpatient surgery. The thread connecting all these specialties was our patients' anxieties, fears, losses, grief and turmoil—their mental health. In 2007, I educated 15 women's health nurses in evidence-based aromatherapy and we developed the first hospital obstetric nursing unit aromatherapy program in the US.

In 2010, with patient data to support the effectiveness of aromatherapy, we received a grant to complete a year-long postpartum depression and anxiety aromatherapy pilot study (Conrad and Adams 2012). The results indicated statistically significant improvement with aromatherapy treatments for both anxiety and depression. The tools used for measuring pre- and post-treatment anxiety and depression were the General Anxiety Disorder 7 (GAD7) (Spitzer *et al.* 2006) and Edinburgh Postnatal Depression Scale (EPDS). The treatments were simple and economically feasible in a clinical or personal setting to help this all too common and at times devastating condition.

In 2018, Singing Dragon publishers contacted me to propose

that I write a women's health evidence-based aromatherapy guidebook for practitioners. This was published in 2019 and has been globally well received by practitioners in the trenches as well as by women for their own self-care.

In the past three years, the world has changed dramatically with unforeseen collective global loss, isolation and devastation to individuals, families, healthcare professionals, economies and mental health. In this guidebook, my goal is to demonstrate the evidence base for the use of aromatherapy in women's mental health and provide you with the tools and specific knowledge about how to create and provide this therapy safely and effectively.

Respect for the evidence base to guide our safest, most well-informed practice will be the focus of this book, which is laced with years of clinical experience, case studies and practical tips to keep the information within easy reach for the majority.

The book will focus on women's mental health and aromatherapy, and I wish to encourage any and all individuals who relate in any way to mental health or aromatherapy, regardless of gender identity, to explore, experiment and enjoy any relevant content to enhance your journey. Utilizing the specific essential oils and methods as shared via the available human evidence base and years of clinical experience provides you with the safest, most effective and economical information. Pregnancy, infants, young children and those with allergies require special considerations.

As in all my work, I encourage you to start with your own self-care and then share with others in your care.

Stay well!

CHAPTER I

Historical Separation of Body, Mind and Spirit

How mental health was sent to the hillside

It all came together in graduate school at Westminster University in London as my professor reviewed the history of our separation—not church and state, but body and mind. This stunning history had never been taught in my US nursing curriculum as it had in Europe and the UK and hearing it was a tremendous moment of enlightenment. In summary, prior to the scientific revolution, the Roman Catholic church had complete control of all aspects of human beings. Since the church forbade and criminalized dissection of the body, individuals were unaware of human anatomy. However, even though it was forbidden, the anatomical accuracy of some Renaissance artists indicates that dissection occurred. In the 1600s, the dawn of scientific inquiry, the church permitted male scientists and physicians solely the right to dissect the human body for scientific exploration, discovery and advancement of knowledge, and the church maintained control and influence of the mind and soul. Recognizing aberrant behaviors and melancholy as illnesses, "therapeutic asylums" emerged to remove potentially dangerous individuals from society.

The study of the mind and emotions emerged as a distinct medical discipline in the early 19th century with Benjamin Rush, the founding father of psychiatry, Sigmund Freud's psychoanalysis and others, thus separating treatment of the mind from the body, while the soul remained the domain of the church. The separation continued in Western medicine until the later part of the 20th century with the advent of integrative and complementary alternative medicine as people suffering from stress, side-effects from treatments for serious health conditions and spiritual voids sought realms beyond allopathic traditional medicine. Previously unimaginable medical feats, such as lifesaving heart and organ transplant surgeries or cancer treatments prolonging lives of children and adults, carried with them unanticipated emotional, spiritual and physical effects. The somewhat underground quest emerged for remedies and modalities outside of the Western medical realm for healing. Aromatherapy, much like music, art and meditation, enters the unseen realm: the "Space of Healing." Perhaps sophisticated scientific tools do not yet fully exist to measure this "Space of Healing"; for the sake of this book, we'll take a leap forward with aromatherapy and emotional health to envision the potential of this amazing aromatic tool to accompany us in our healing.

CHAPTER 2

Aromatherapy

A Complementary Therapy

Aromatherapy is a descendant of herbal medicine, the oldest form of healing on the planet. Essential oils, the tools of aromatherapy, are steam distillates of aromatic plants or, in the case of citrus oils, they're cold pressed. The complex chemistry of individual oils creates the unique scents and provides the therapeutic properties utilized for clinical treatments and home remedies. Plants yield different amounts of oil, which is the reason for the range of costs between oils. For example, lavender produces a much greater quantity of oil per plant than rose, which is much more expensive. Mother Nature's bounty of flowers, barks, needles, leaves, fruits, buds and seeds all produce essential oils. The oils are very concentrated; as an example, it has been widely shared that 1 drop of peppermint oil equals 28 tea bags of plant material, so not much is needed to have a positive effect. Too much can be overpowering and if overused, can increase individuals' sensitivities or cause skin irritations or burns, so care is advised. When focusing on mental health, with the aim of affecting one's emotions so they feel better, the method of use is most often direct or indirect inhalation of the oil; this is the quickest route and effective for reducing anxiety states and uplifting mood. Long regarded in modern times as a stress reduction therapy, it is pleasantly scented, simple to use, painless and economical when used appropriately; it doesn't require a prescription, and is readily available and ideal for self-care. In most instances, while respecting allergies and personal preferences, mental health toolkits are enhanced with aromatherapy. Regardless of the complexity of the condition—from situational anxiety or mild depression to schizophrenia or bipolar illness—anyone can benefit from pleasant therapeutic scents to improve how they're feeling and lessen their suffering. External use assures safety if used correctly and there are virtually no contraindications or drug interactions when used alongside prescription medication, which is ideal for the wide range and severity of mental health conditions and treatments. Homes, clinics, hospitals, offices or institutional settings can be enhanced and less intimidating; we'll explore evidence and practice-based essential oils and methods suitable for various conditions and environments.

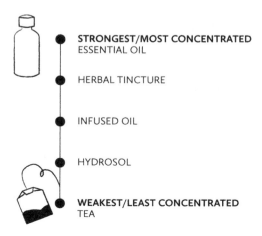

STRONGEST/MOST CONCENTRATED
ESSENTIAL OIL

HERBAL TINCTURE

INFUSED OIL

HYDROSOL

WEAKEST/LEAST CONCENTRATED
TEA

CHAPTER 3

Women's Mental Health

History

The intriguing history of mental health and women ranged from magical beliefs of evil spirit possession to inhumane and extreme surgical procedures to experiment with, enhance or alter misunderstood female anatomy. In addition, Hippocrates "the father of medicine," labeled female emotional conditions "hysteria," with the belief that they originated from abnormal movements of the uterus in the body (Tasca *et al.* 2012) and/or lack of sexual relations with males. It was believed at the time that childbirth could lead to a "sad uterus" and accompanying physical and emotional anomalies. Moral reckoning cast by clergy, guilt for infertility, melancholy, and an overall lack of scientific knowledge, education and personal control of one's own body negatively altered the lives of thousands of women through the ages. Lobotomies and ECT "shock treatments" for the most serious cases were common among the institutionalized.

The dawn of psychiatric medications in the pharmaceutical industry introduced antipsychotic, antidepressant and numbing anti-anxiety medications, such as Valium and Librium, which were widely prescribed to women naive of their addictive potential. In the 1980s, the diagnosis of hysterical neurosis was finally removed from the DSM, the diagnostic manual for mental health practitioners. Barbara Gordon offers a personal account of Valium addiction and reveals the overprescribing of anti-anxiety medications as "happy pills" by physicians for women with anxiety, stress and overall dissatisfaction in life in *I'm Dancing as Fast as I Can* (Gordon 1979). In 1990, as a graduate psychiatric nursing student writing a psychopharmacology paper, I was referred to a neurologist for tingling in my lips, hands and feet. Having recently read the book for class, I was shocked when, without reading my history or conducting a standard neurological exam, the neurologist prescribed Valium and stated, "Just take these and you won't care about anything, hide them in your purse, don't even tell your husband." Shocked and insulted, I respectfully challenged and declined the prescription. I expressed the reason for the referral appointment— the possibility of multiple sclerosis as my age and my symptoms aligned with this—and also shared my recently acquired psychiatric nursing graduate school knowledge about physicians inappropriately prescribing addictive medications for women without even conducting a neurological exam, and the consultation ended abruptly. Ultimately, nerve compression in my neck from an earlier whiplash injury exacerbated by musculoskeletal changes from a recent pregnancy was identified as the cause of my symptoms by a female osteopath who listened to her patient and practiced holistic medicine. I'll always believe the timing of this incident guided my understanding of other women's experiences with male physicians, a bit of valuable indoctrination which also continued my trajectory into viewing humans as whole, with each experience and injury affecting the whole being: the mind–body connection. It's understandable that women have trust issues with male physicians and choose to self-treat and to care for those in their nurturing space with remedies such as aromatherapy.

Data and statistics

According to the Centers for Disease Control and Prevention (2022a):

> **Mental health** includes our emotional, psychological, and social well-being. It affects how we think, feel, and act. It also helps determine how we handle stress, relate to others, and make choices. Mental health is important at every stage of life, from childhood and adolescence through adulthood.

Mental health in the US

According to the National Alliance on Mental Illness (NAMI) (2022):

- 1 in 5 US adults experience mental illness each year, with women experiencing many conditions at a rate greater than men.

- 1 in 20 US adults experience serious mental illness each year.

- 1 in 6 US youths aged 6–17 experience a mental health disorder each year.

- 50% of all lifetime mental illness begins by age 14, and 75% by age 24.

According to the National Institute of Mental Health (NIMH 2022a):

- In 2020, there were an estimated 52.9 million adults aged 18 or older in the United States with AMI (Any Mental Illness). This number represented 21% of all US adults.

- The prevalence of AMI was higher among females (25.8%) than males (15.8%).

- Young adults aged 18–25 years had the highest prevalence of AMI (30.6%) compared to adults aged 26–49 years (25.3%) and aged 50 and older (14.5%).

- The prevalence of AMI was highest among the adults reporting two or more races (35.8%), followed by white adults (22.6%). The prevalence of AMI was lowest among Asian adults (13.9%).

Mental health globally

According to the World Health Organization (WHO 2022), the COVID-19 pandemic triggered a 25 percent increase in prevalence of anxiety and depression worldwide:

- Anxiety: As of March 2022, 27% of US adults reported symptoms of anxiety, with the highest rate in the past two years of 37% in November 2021.

- Depression: As of March 2022, 21.7% of US adults reported symptoms of depression, with the highest rate in the past two years at 30.2% in December 2020.

Mental health in women

According to the US Office on Women's Health (2021):

- More than 1 in 5 women in the United States experienced a mental health condition.

- In 2020, there were around 15.49 million families with a female householder and no spouse present in the United States.

- In the United States, about 43.6% of women and 24.8% of men experienced some form of sexual violence in their lifetime, according to the National Intimate Partner and Sexual Violence Survey (Centers for Disease Control and Prevention (CDC) 2016/2017). About 21.3% of women surveyed reported completed or attempted rape at some point in their lives.

- Infertility, the inability to conceive after one year of unprotected sex, affects 10–15% of couples in the United States.

- Financially, women make an average 20% less money than men.

Some mental health conditions affect more women than men. Women are more likely to suffer from the following types of mental health issues:

Major depressive disorder

According to the National Institute of Mental Health (NIMH 2022b), major depression is one of the most common mental disorders in the United States.

According to the Anxiety and Depression Association of America (ADAA 2022), major depressive disorder affects more than 16.1 million American adults. Research indicates that major depressive episodes are more common among adult females than adult males.

Generalized anxiety disorder (GAD)
Another common women's mental health issue is anxiety. According to ADAA (2022), GAD affects 6.8 million adults in the US. Women are twice as likely to be affected by GAD than men, and it is also common for women to have both depression and anxiety.

Post-traumatic stress disorder (PTSD)
PTSD affects 7.7 million adults in the US. Women are more likely to be affected than men, in part because PTSD is often triggered by traumatic experiences that are more common in women (NIMH 2022c).

Conditions and disorders specific to females
While people of different genders can struggle with most mental disorders, there are some conditions that can only affect individuals assigned female at birth. These disorders are specific to females due to hormones and the ability to carry and give birth to children. There are three common disorders specific to females:

- **Premenstrual syndrome** (PMS) and **premenstrual dysphoric disorder** (PMDD): Symptoms are irritability, depression, or anxiety in the week or two before a menstrual period begins. PMDD is similar to PMS, but with more severe symptoms and is a more serious, debilitating condition.

- **Postpartum depression:** Postpartum depression goes beyond the "baby blues" most women experience in the days after giving birth. Symptoms include feeling hopeless, empty and sad. The most severe is **postpartum psychosis**, a rare, very serious psychiatric condition that occurs in 1 in 1000 births (Jones 2020).

- **Perimenopausal depression:** As women transition to menopause (a period called perimenopause), their risk of depression increases. The declining levels of estrogen during this time may bring on depression. Guidelines for diagnosing and treating this type of depression are very new.

Women are more likely to seek help for certain conditions

According to *Psychology Today,* one in four women will seek treatment for mental health at some point, compared to only one in ten men (Young 2015).

Statistics in most realms of mental health indicate a higher likelihood of conditions amongst females. Historically, a range of biological, economic, educational and social circumstances have all contributed to this reality. Until recently, females lacked the educational opportunities for advancement and thus self-actualization, realization of dreams, satisfaction and financial independence. Societal and familial expectations of the female role, with minimal role models, thwarted dreams and full realization of intellectual, athletic and leadership gifts. Negative messaging about women commonly heard in my childhood from males, and at times jealous or judgmental females, included: "She has a mind of her own," "She thinks for herself," "She thinks she's all that," "Who wears the pants in the family?" "She sure does speak her own mind," "She was a bad girl," "If she just kept her legs closed," and "She got what she deserved," not to mention how the names given solely to females for assertiveness in communication, intimate relations or goal achievement have all affected the collective female sense of self.

Significant programming led to a collective sense of females somehow being less than males, second-class citizens, never quite enough, and that they should be sure to not be too much or outshine them—over time this mixed messaging, fear, shame and guilt has chipped away at women's mental health. Eating disorders and self-harm behaviors are much more common in females and speak to the extreme measures of dealing with trauma, self-loathing, depression and anxiety. Historically, non-white females experienced additional hurdles of less access to quality educational, healthcare, reproductive, financial and housing services, and leadership opportunities than their white counterparts.

In my high school, as the tides began to shift, two cheerleaders and gymnasts in long-term relationships became pregnant; they were immediately removed from the cheerleading squad, gymnastic team and school, while their male athlete boyfriends were permitted to remain on their teams and stayed in school without any repercussions. The girls, strengthened by family and friends, fought the school board to win their right to remain in school and judge cheerleading tryouts; it was the first time girls fought and remained in school in our Midwest city and possibly state. Fortunately, decades later, I can share that both strong and intelligent women have thrived, married, and have had additional children and successful careers; one remains married and the other is in a successful second marriage. Most probably these incidents strengthened their resolve to face life's challenges and demonstrated to the rest of us that we had a right to fight for equality in even the most difficult and public circumstances. Understandably, far too many young girls lack the familial, cultural and group support and resources to stand up for themselves, leaving them at an early disadvantage educationally, financially and socially. Early experiences can chip away at a woman's self-confidence and self-worth and can unfortunately diminish opportunities for the life she dreamt of, imagined and deserved, leading to higher risks of mental health conditions.

A world of unrealistic expectations of "Barbie doll" physical beauty created a world of eating disorders, plastic surgery, cultural disparity, unrealistic postpartum bodies and unhealthy concepts of natural aging that have taken a huge toll on the female psyche. When striving to attain personal and professional goals, an expected pregnancy may negatively impact a female's educational and career opportunities, financial freedom and ultimately the woman's mental health. All of this contributes significantly to women's struggles with mental health.

In addition, females are more likely than males to seek treatment for themselves and their families as well as have increased exposure to medical professionals during pregnancies, childbirth and menopause, providing a pool of data to better understand physical and emotional health patterns amongst females. Cyclical monthly hormonal and neurotransmitter level alterations with accompanying physical and emotional symptoms highlight clear physiological differences in females which give rise to unique mental health challenges. As cited throughout the guidebook, evidence highlights aromatherapy's positive effects on women's emotional wellbeing —a valuable tool for self-care.

Reproductive rights, healthcare access and mental health repercussions

In the last week of June 2022, a major shift occurred in women's reproductive rights with the US Supreme court overturning the 50-year-old Roe vs Wade legal abortion law. This catapults most women in reproductive age to greater uncertainty about the future of their birth control options, availability, privacy, trust, safety and beyond. The 50 states will have laws ranging from safe and legal medical and pharmaceutical services in some states to banned, illegal and potentially criminal services in other states, setting women back decades. Women with limited financial resources, familial support, transportation and proximity to gynecological or prenatal clinical care will suffer the most. This most certainly will affect the mental health, the already rising anxiety, depression and panic, of so many women with concerns for themselves and their children.

Life Stages and Emotional Challenges

Mental Health Issues During Women's Reproductive Years

Late teens–young adults

Alarming rates of suicide in teens and young adults, our personal and societal treasures, have led to increased focus on outreach mental health programs in schools, communities and society at large. The isolation caused by the pandemic wreaked havoc on the social fiber of traditional passages such as proms, graduations, university admissions and musical and athletic performances, as well as the critical daily social rhythm of young people's lives, growth and development. Stigma, access, privacy and cost are hurdles that can prevent many from obtaining necessary medical or psychological treatment. Complementary therapies, specifically aromatherapy, offer a pleasant and readily accessible tool to ease emotional distress, at least in the short term. If at all possible, an evaluation by a medical or psychological professional is of utmost importance, particularly with major depression, or suicidal or homicidal ideations. Unfortunately, prescribed antidepressant medications take precious time to reach full therapeutic effectiveness, and may have paradoxical unwanted effects or pose undesirable risks. Many people dislike the side-effects and some experience worsening of symptoms, which is not ideal in any way and can be life-threatening in worst-case scenarios.

This is a group where aromatherapy can play a role during the rough patches. It's painless, private, inexpensive and readily available. In practice, we offer a few different oils with known anti-anxiety and/or antidepressant properties to smell for personal preference. The responses are generally immediate, so let them choose and every few weeks switch it up as circumstances, body chemistry, menstrual cycles, appeal and effectiveness change. Encourage them to try different scents, as it's empowering to personally choose one, or even make a blend of 2–4 oils and label with a name, feeling state or theme of preference. In practice, with teens and young adults navigating traumas, divorce, death, fears, challenges at school, focus issues or personal anxieties, a selected oil or personal blend used on their terms as needed in a personal inhaler or room diffuser has smoothed and eased the rough patches and seemed cool to them, and most shared that they loved it.

Studies of mostly female high school and university students demonstrated reduction in stress, anxiety, pain and stress response levels with inhalations of lavender, sandalwood, rose or bergamot or lotion massage with lavender, sweet marjoram and clary sage (Ou *et al.* 2012; Seo *et al.* 2009). Meta-analysis of 15 studies of aromatherapy for agitation and aggression behaviors demonstrated significant improvements in agitation levels with inhalations of lavender over up to four weeks (Xiao *et al.* 2021).

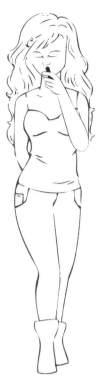

Aromatherapy improves focus, uplifts mood and calms anxiety.

In practice, spritzers of bergamot or ylang-ylang work wonders with the irritability, anger and awkwardness of adolescents. Inhalations of peppermint, rosemary and sweet orange blended in an inhaler or desk diffuser enhance focus, aiding study time. Inhalations on a cotton pad, inhaler or spritzers of mandarin or yuzu uplift and pleasantly ease anxiety. Ten-minute (or ten times) slow, deep inhalations of the "panic oils" frankincense and/or neroli, alone or blended equally on a cotton pad or in a personal inhaler, quickly decrease intense panic-type anxiety. Lavender, rosemary, roman chamomile and sweet marjoram singly or blended in lotion are phenomenal for athletic muscular or menstrual cramps.

In addition to aromatherapy, four drops of homeopathic Bach Flower Rescue Remedy in water or juice four times daily eases stress and is readily available. The flower essences although similar to homeopathy, function more as energy medicine.

There are instances, such as a shock or unexpected bad news, where a one-time inhalation of a single oil calms the individual and gets them through the moment. Other times, such as with cyclical PMS, PMDD, ongoing anxiety, panic and depression, it's important to encourage ongoing use, such as "Inhale this 4x/daily and as needed for 2–3 weeks" to note and experience beneficial changes. With most professional cases, the individual needs the benefit of the oil's therapeutic properties over a period of time to fully assess and experience the effectiveness. Write it out specifically or, if you have the appropriate level of education and certification in aromatherapy and prescriptive authority, prescribe it for them.

As a parent of a teen using aromatherapy for self-care, if they don't choose to share how they're feeling, use of their aromatherapy can be a helpful clue that they're not feeling great or something is going on. Changing the oils or blends every two to three weeks enhances effectiveness as teens' situations, menstrual cycles and needs are frequently changing, which affects their body chemistry and the corresponding oil choices. As a rule, they enjoy this process, especially when they have access to and control of it.

Suicide attempts and aromatherapy

Young people are at particular risk of suicide (CDC 2022b). Full brain maturity isn't complete until 26 years of age and adolescents are prone to impulsivity. Additionally, full understanding of cause and effect, that a current heartbreaking situation will pass, and the absolute finality of death are not complete in teens and young adults. With this emerging science, mental health support and services are clearly needed to protect the greatest and most precious resources: our young people.

Schools, locker rooms, community centers, shelters and outreach programs could implement aromatherapy to decrease agitation, irritability and anxiety or uplift depressive moods. Emotions are undeniably altered while listening to music, escaping into a painting, smelling bread baking, receiving a massage or a hug, or in the week before their period eases emotional and physical upheaval.

In higher-risk and medically underserved areas, the potential for novel programs is endless. With data on increased productivity in Japan's workplaces with lemon diffusion (Ipek 2004), anecdotal decreases in aggressive behavior in psychiatric centers with lavender diffusion, and increases in department store sales with citrus scents, there's potential for positive emotional responses with aromatherapy. These behaviors and feelings are all reminders of the power of our senses and their often under-appreciated potential in emotional health and healing. Studies and practice experience indicate that females are more sensitive than males to scents, particularly at certain times in the menstrual cycle as well as during pregnancy. Encouraging young women to experiment with a few different scents helps determine what appeals and will be most therapeutic for them.

In public or open areas, it's also important to be respectful of others' allergies and/or asthma and provide scent-free areas. Single essential oils, rather than blends with multiple oils, are the least complicated and have shown effectiveness. Citrus oils rarely provoke allergic reactions, are familiar and universally pleasant. For some people, the memory of florals or strong scents may cause emotional reactions when they are exposed to them; while lavender, the most popular essential oil, and chamomile can exacerbate asthma and seasonal allergies for some individuals.

Amadeo and colleagues' fascinating six-month pilot suicide prevention study (2020) included the addition of aromatherapy massage with 10 percent ylang-ylang essential oil to traditional medical and psychological treatments. Study results demonstrated that individuals who received four aromatherapy treatments in four months of the six-month study had significantly fewer suicide attempts than the traditional psychiatric treatment only control group. The combination included initial psychiatric evaluation, ongoing follow-up telephone calls and postcards, combining touch via professional massage and the pharmacological properties of ylang-ylang both inhaled and applied through skin absorption. Ylang-ylang, which is indigenous and familiar to individuals in the study location, is well known for strong anxiolytic/anxiety-reducing effect. Results indicated significantly reduced numbers of suicide attempts and suicide (3%) in the aromatherapy massage group at six months compared with the control group (12%). The combination of touch, smell, professional communication and crisis-call availability highlights the value of multifaceted therapies in the treatment of severe depression and suicide. It's impossible to avoid highlighting the gap in human connection and caring. This study is filled with the combination of skilled talk therapies, touch via massage and the pleasant pharmacologically calming and uplifting properties of ylang-ylang essential oil.

> Ylang-ylang, a strong floral scent, can cause headaches and though the 10 percent dilution was clearly effective and probably necessary in Amadeo *et al.*'s study, a much stronger scent may be unpleasant.

Premenstrual syndrome

Data confirms that the incidence of anxiety and depressive disorders and/or treatment-seeking for these conditions is greater among biological females than males (Altemus, Saravaya and Epperson 2014). In the reproductive years, spanning 40 or more years, females' monthly fluctuating hormone levels produce a 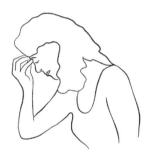 wide range of physical and emotional symptoms from relatively mild to severe. Premenstrual syndrome (PMS), which affects 30–80 percent of women of reproductive age (ADAA 2023), is a series of unpleasant physical and emotional symptoms occurring from mid-cycle to menses/start of bleeding and is diagnosed based on the timing of the symptoms in relation to the menstrual cycle. Premenstrual dysphoric disorder (PMDD), a psychiatric diagnosis, is the most severe form of this condition, with increased irritability, depression and anxiety affecting the ability to function normally, often requiring prescribed medication. The mechanisms causing these conditions are not fully understood, but recent studies highlight the potential interplay and sensitivity of the neurotransmitters GABA (gamma-aminobutyric acid) and serotonin and the fluctuation of the sexual hormones, progesterone and estrogen. Serotonin and GABA at normal levels have a positive effect by promoting relaxation, uplifted mood and a general sense of wellbeing. When the neurotransmitter levels are decreased, this wreaks havoc on the emotions, leading to irritability, mood swings, anxiety, panic and depression to varying degrees. In some women, this reality can occur for 7–10 days *every month,* clearly interfering with school, work, extracurricular activities, performance and relationships. Exercise, diet and supplementation have been shown to ease the symptoms and the more severe cases are often prescribed selective serotonin reuptake inhibitors (SSRIs), the most common antidepressants. For many, these medications have unpleasant side-effects and in young adults can pose risks of worsening depression. In some cases suicides have been blamed on them, so they now carry a black box warning; hardly an ideal treatment (Fornaro *et al.* 2019; Ho 2012; Teicher *et al.* 1990).

An interplay exists between hormone and neurotransmitter (NT) levels—when they are out of balance women's PMS symptoms are often more severe. Human and animal studies confirm that estrogen and progesterone hormone receptors in key areas of the brain are in close proximity and interwoven with neurotransmitters that affect emotions and mental health. As estrogen and progesterone levels fluctuate in the monthly menstrual cycle, this triggers the GABAergic (the main inhibitory and calming NT) and serotoninergic (the main NT associated with depression) neurotransmitters, leading to increases in anxiety, anger, irritability and depressive symptoms.

Aromatherapy and PMS emotional symptoms

Aromatherapy is well known as an overall stress management therapy as it reduces anxiety, fear and panic and instills a sense of calm. Most earlier studies measured pre/post individual responses to aromatherapy interventions. Recently, by exploring the mechanisms of these actions on an in-depth cellular, neurotransmitter, hormonal and physiological level, studies are providing important data for therapeutic actions and potential treatment opportunities in women's health. Methodology and frequency are also important therapeutic considerations. In our practice, PMS aromatherapy interventions are twice-daily lotion blend applications starting 10 days prior to the menstrual period until the onset or first 1–2 days of bleeding, that is, the *luteal phase*. This corresponds directly with the changes in hormonal and neurotransmitter levels.

The constituents of essential oils that produce sedative, anxiolytic and antidepressant effects in various studies, often appear to be interacting with the GABAergic system (Costa *et al.* 2011; Granger *et al.* 2005; Koo *et al.* 2004; Van Brederode *et al.* 2016; Wang and Heinbockel 2018). A noteworthy exception is lavender (*lavandula angustifolia*), by far the most studied essential oil, which indicates strong anxiolytic/anti-anxiety effects in multiple studies. Chioca *et al.* (2013) indicated that lavender probably exerted its anxiolytic effects through the serotonergic, not GABA, system.

The safety, effectiveness, availability and affordability of aromatherapy make it an ideal option for the majority of women. Young women and teens are particularly vulnerable to PMS and to the side-effects of the medications, such as SSRIs, prescribed to treat them. In addition, access to and affordability of healthcare can be stumbling blocks for treatment. Essential oils, the tools of aromatherapy, are readily available in health food stores, pharmacies and online. Even though a woman may choose an essential oil company with membership fees, there are many well-established companies with excellent oils and great clinical reputations that do not require the extra financial or time involvement (see Resources section). Minimal amounts are needed for each treatment and generally the duration of PMS is 7–10 days, the luteal phase of the cycle before bleeding starts, so it only requires twice-daily treatments on those specific days, then treatment can be discontinued until the next month.

Highlights of PMS aromatherapy studies (N = # of people in the study)

A meta-analysis and systematic review of eight qualifying PMS aromatherapy studies collectively demonstrated decreases in anxiety, depression, fatigue, overall PMS scores and psychological symptoms (Es-haghee *et al.* 2020). In a related systematic review of rose oil and menstrual symptoms, Koohpayeh *et al.* (2021) demonstrate similar improvements.

- Geethanjali *et al.* (2020) N = 60: Inhalation of clary sage in water for 20 minutes.

- Heydari *et al.* (2018a, 2018b, 2019) each study with N = 64–66: Women inhaled either neroli 0.5, rose 4% or both twice daily for five days.

- Lotfipur-Rafsanjani *et al.* (2018) study N = 75: Women self-massaged with geranium 2% 30 minutes twice weekly for two weeks.

- Matsumoto *et al.* (2016) studies N = 17: Diffuser with lavender or yuzu.

- Uzunçakmak and Alkaya (2018) study N = 77: Lavender steam inhalation 5 sessions/cycle.

- Koohpayeh *et al.* (2021): Effects of *Rosa damascena* (Damask rose) on menstruation-related pain, headache, fatigue, anxiety, and bloating and an overlapping physical and emotional menstrual aromatherapy meta-analysis demonstrating improvement: A systematic review and meta-analysis of randomized controlled trials.

When treating PMS, timing and frequency are critical to success. Twice daily is very effective and compliance is good with morning and evening routines. In addition to twice daily, women with more acute distress may use the treatments as needed. Most women are familiar with the onset and pattern of their symptoms, so it is best to start the aromatherapy at the first physical or emotional signal and continue until menses/bleeding begins, and for some through days one to two. As the hormone levels change with the start of the period so do the PMS symptoms. With the majority, once menses begins, there's no need to continue until symptoms emerge the following month, so if the cycle is very regular, it's close to 2.5 weeks off, 1.5 weeks on. As with most natural therapies for PMS, three consecutive months are encouraged to fully evaluate the effectiveness of the aromatherapy. Fortunately, with many, we've noted improvement in the first month, which inspires women to continue the aromatherapy routine.

With PMDD, the more severe form of PMS, continue monthly until symptoms improve; the woman always knows when she feels better. This may continue for many months and can then be used as needed. The beauty of aromatherapy for PMS is the cyclical nature which, by design, provides a pause in the treatment, a wash-out per se, increasing the likelihood of ongoing effectiveness. Oftentimes women find the scent of the selected PMS oils unpleasant or even repulsive when not in the luteal phase, which is a helpful assessment tool they can use to determine the timing if their cycle is not regular.

Clinical practice tip

Multiple PMS aromatherapy studies have shown statistically significant improved emotional and physical symptoms after regular 1–2x daily inhalations or skin applications/massage of single or blended essential oils of neroli, rose, lavender, yuzu, geranium, ylang-ylang and clary sage during the luteal phase.

Quick reference table: Aromatherapy for PMS

Condition	Essential oils	Methods
Anxiety	Lavender, rose, neroli, yuzu, geranium, clary sage	Inhalation, diffuser, steam inhalation, self-massage, massage

Depression	Lavender, rose, neroli, yuzu, geranium, clary sage	Inhalation, diffuser, steam inhalation
Fatigue	Rose	Inhalation, self-massage, massage
Irritability	Rose, ylang-ylang, clary sage, geranium, neroli, lavender	Inhalation, self-massage
Anger	Ylang-ylang, rose	Inhalation, self-massage
Physical symptoms: bloating, edema, pain	Rose, geranium, lavender	Self-massage, massage, footbath

Pregnancy and anxiety

Along with joy, for many, pregnancy produces feelings of concern, fear, uncertainty, anxiety and obsession about the developing baby and the role of motherhood. Anxiety is common in the first trimester as women adjust to the reality of pregnancy and often feel unwell, or traumatized by previous losses, and also between 18 and 32 weeks, which coincides with fetal developmental screening tests (Bastard and Tiran 2005). In past generations, motherhood was expected, difficult to prevent and the primary role for a married woman. Convents were the only respectable alternative—women living together, married to Jesus, with strict rules where women, perhaps with a spiritual calling, could avoid the traditional roles of wife and mother and instead fulfill intellectual, academic and service roles. Modern women with personal and financial independence, choices for partnering and satisfying careers often delay or consider avoiding pregnancy for fear of losing themselves or all they've worked so hard to attain; others experience fertility challenges. In many women, any and all of these scenarios fused with familial and social expectations intensify anxiety, guilt, depression, shame and grief. Establishing trust is paramount for openly exploring a woman's range of past experiences, fears, doubts and personal choices. Aromatherapy gently and surprisingly enters spaces for therapeutic communication and emotional release of long-held or immediate concerns. In a clinical setting, pleasant scents as a therapeutic tool transcend physical, emotional and historic client expectations. Thus, much like a gift, appreciation and a sense of wellbeing arise in the therapeutic relationship.

Studies indicate that scent memories can intensify anxiety, so incorporating questions regarding positive and negative memories provides guidance for aromatherapy options. With significant hormonal shifts in pregnancy, the intertwined senses of smell and taste are often intensified and altered. Fortunately, the aversion to stronger scents in pregnancy aligns perfectly with the prenatal aromatherapy evidence base of safe and effective 1% dilutions. Prenatal evaluations for mental and emotional health such as the most utilized EPDS (Edinburgh Postpartum Depression Scale), HADS (Hospital Anxiety Depression Scale) and BDI (Beck Depression Inventory, Beck *et al.* 1988) are valuable tools to identify women at risk for prenatal and postpartum depression. They're easy to administer and score in the office while awaiting the physician or midwife. Early identification and follow-up of women with potential increased risks for depression provide practitioner opportunities for education and early intervention, including aromatherapy. Clinically, I have found that treating women with a history or increased risk of depression throughout pregnancy/postpartum decreases the incidence of postpartum depression. Selection of essential oils with antidepressant uplifting properties are recommended in these cases.

There are several standardized easy-to-administer anxiety screening tools, such as the:

* Spielberger Trait Anxiety Inventory (STAI)

* Generalized Anxiety Disorder Assessment (GAD7)

* Beck Anxiety Inventory (BAI).

Tocophobia is a severe fear of pregnancy and childbirth requiring therapy. Aromatherapy used alongside can help ease the anxiety. These women may need a variety of therapies throughout their pregnancy and a trusted therapist, obstetrics (OB) nurse, midwife or doula would provide a comprehensive team of support. Inhalations, personal inhalers, room sprays or diffusers offer a soft calming atmosphere to decrease escalation of anxiety and fears and are supportive to both the woman and developing babe.

Quick reference table: Prenatal evidence-based aromatherapy

Condition	Essential oils	Methods*
Anxiety	Lavender, petitgrain, bergamot, neroli	Inhalation, diffusion, footbath, massage 1% after 16 weeks
Depression	Lavender, petitgrain, bergamot, lemon, peppermint, neroli	Inhalation, diffuser, spritzer 1% after 16 weeks

Condition	Essential oils	Methods*
Fear	Lavender, neroli, bergamot, petitgrain	Inhalation or diffuser 1%
Panic	Neroli	Inhalation
Irritability	Lavender, bergamot, neroli	Inhalation
Pain	Lavender, peppermint	Footbath, massage, inhalation 1%
Sleep	Lavender	Footbath, inhalation, massage 1%
Stress	Lavender, bergamot, petitgrain, lemon	Inhalation, diffuser, footbath, massage 1%

1 percent dilution, the recommended amount during pregnancy, is created by adding 1 drop of essential oil to 5 ml/1 tsp lotion or carrier oil.

Postpartum depression

The time after childbirth—from six weeks to one year, depending on one's culture—is defined as the postpartum period. The joyful bliss of motherhood depicted in magazines and television often misrepresents many women's true feelings. Overwhelmed with the new role, significant body alterations and hormonal 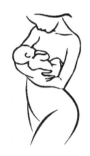 upheaval, many experience sadness and an unexpected loss of sense of self. In the first 48–72 hours, as hormone levels adjust, most women experience a short period of "baby blues" with tears and sadness, which passes within a few days. According to multiple studies, one in 7–10 women experience postpartum depression, with feelings ranging from depression, anxiety and lack of interest in the baby to the rare and most serious postpartum psychosis, a loss of touch with reality. Often unexpected, these experiences, which are so far from the expected fluffy pink and blue maternal bliss, blindside the woman and her spouse/partner, ushering in a host of unforeseen personal and familial stresses in addition to adapting to the role as parent. Guilt, shame and fear prevent some from sharing their feelings or seeking treatment. Multiple studies demonstrate the benefit of aromatherapy inhalations or massages, which can significantly decrease depression and anxiety. Conrad and Adams (2012), in a one-year high-risk postpartum study at four-week intervals, demonstrated statistically significant improvements in both anxiety GAD7 and depression EPDS results in the aromatherapy group with 10-minute, twice weekly 2 percent lavender and rose inhalations or hand massages. Kianpour *et al.*'s (2018) 38-week prenatal to six weeks postpartum study found that 10 deep inhalations of rosewater and lavender at bedtime significantly decreased depression. Kianpour *et al.*'s (2016) postpartum depression study with inhalations every eight hours of lavender for four weeks significantly decreased postpartum depression. In Chile, our postpartum depression clinic midwifery aromatherapy case series demonstrated significant reduction in depression EPDS scores with daily spritzer and inhalations of mandarin and lemon for 40 days. Chen *et al.*'s (2022) study in Taiwan demonstrated that 15-minute daily bergamot inhalations in a postpartum center significantly decreased depression EPDS. All these studies utilized readily available essential oils via regularly timed simple inhalations for four to six week durations with positive results.

Quick postpartum depression facts and statistics[1]

- Approximately 1 in 10 women will experience post-partum depression after giving birth, with some studies reporting 1 in 7 women.

- Postpartum depression generally lasts three to six months, however, this varies based on several factors. "Based on research and conversations with postpartum professionals and specialists, many women don't seek help until 12–18 months postpartum" (personal communication with Birdie Meyer, past president of PSI Postpartum Support International).

- It is estimated that nearly 50% of mothers with post-partum depression are not diagnosed by a health professional. This is an opportunity for aromatherapists to treat and refer to mental health professionals.

- 80% of women with postpartum depression will achieve a full recovery.

Quick reference table: Postpartum evidence-based oils

Condition	Essential oils (up to three in a blend)	Methods
Anxiety	Rose, lavender, neroli, frankincense, mandarin, ylang-ylang, sweet marjoram	Inhalation, shoulder or hand massage
Baby blues	Rose, jasmine, lavender, mandarin, sweet orange, lemon, bergamot, neroli	Inhalation, shoulder or hand massage, spritzer

1   See www.postpartumdepression.org/resources/statistics

Depression	Rose, jasmine, lavender, neroli, mandarin, sweet orange, lemon, bergamot, petitgrain	Inhalation on cotton pad or inhaler, spritzer, diffuser, massage, bath
Fear	Rose, frankincense, geranium, lavender	Spritzer, inhalation, footbath, shoulder or hand massage
Fatigue	Lemon, sweet orange, jasmine, peppermint (if not around infant)	Inhalation, spritzer
Grief	Frankincense, rose, lavender, mandarin, peppermint	Spritzer, inhalation on cotton pad, blanket spray
Insomnia	Lavender, mandarin, Roman chamomile	Inhalation, spritzer on sheets
Irritability	Ylang-ylang, rose, clary sage, geranium	Inhalation, spritzer or shoulder massage
Panic	Frankincense, rose, neroli	Inhalation
Stress	Lavender, rose, geranium, neroli, frankincense, ylang-ylang	Inhalation, shoulder or hand massage

Perimenopause

Perimenopause, the stage before menopause, usually begins in the 40s (unless
surgical menopause from a total hysterectomy occurs) and, in some women, can
last up to ten years. This stage can trigger
a range of emotions from fear of aging,
anxiety about the future and depression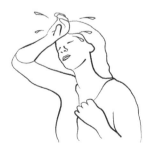
about losing fertility and youthfulness. It can involve physi-
cal changes affecting intimacy, painful intercourse, changing

sexual desire and grief for loss of attractiveness and the beauty of youth, or a feeling of becoming invisible in society. Rose, the "queen of flowers," eases anxiety and depression in this stage and is an appealing scent at this stage of life. In our women's health practice, I've observed that the scent of rose oil is generally preferred by women 45+ with the exception of during PMS, labor and early postpartum, which seems to indicate a potential hormonal influence.

As hormone levels, particularly estrogen, decline, symptoms vary. Menopause is defined as one consecutive year without a menstrual period and on average occurs at 51 years of age. Estrogen levels progressively decrease, wreaking havoc on many women. Vasomotor symptoms of hot flashes and night sweats, insomnia, tachycardia ("racing heart"), vaginal dryness and atrophy, and emotional lability are all common symptoms. Highs and lows, anxiety and depression, frame this stage of many women's lives. Monthly menstrual cycles and fertility are finished for the remainder of their lives. Initially many women celebrate this time, particularly if heavy bleeding, cramps, moodiness and/or the financial strain of monthly menstrual supplies were a burden. Over time, for many, the reality of ending this unique and defining aspect of being a woman—sexuality, pregnancy, infertility, losses, femininity, and then the reality of aging—creeps into consciousness. Anxiety, depression and feeling something has changed affect a woman's mental health. In Western society, certainly in the US, the subtle and not so subtle negative menopausal messaging of diminished femininity and attractiveness and less value as a person insidiously chips away at many women's psyche. Honest, open and empowering communication facilitates understanding of the very real physiological changes occurring; the resulting physical and emotional effects coupled with internal voices, as well as ancestral and societal influences, challenge emotional wellbeing and mental health.

Quick reference table: Aromatherapy for perimenopause–menopause

Condition	Essential oils	Methods
Anxiety	Rose, lavender, geranium, neroli, ylang-ylang, yuzu	Inhalation on cotton pad or personal inhaler, diffuser, spritzer
Depression	Lavender, rose, jasmine, geranium, bergamot, mandarin	Inhalation on cotton pad or personal inhaler, diffuser, spritzer
Irritability	Ylang-ylang, neroli, geranium, lavender, clary sage	Inhalation, shoulder or hand massage
Intimacy/ sexual desire/ relaxation	Jasmine, rose, lavender, ylang-ylang, fennel, geranium, neroli	Inhalation, couple's massages, room or sheet spritzer
Grief	Rose, lavender, frankincense	Inhalation, massage
"Racing heart"/ tachycardia	Ylang-ylang	Inhalation on cotton pad, diffuser. *Always have evaluated by a medical doctor*
Difficulty concentrating/ focusing	Rosemary, peppermint, lemon	Inhalation on pad, diffuser, spritzer
Mood changes	Geranium, clary sage, rose, ylang-ylang	Inhalation, skin application on shoulders, chest, wrists

Post-menopause–old age

Emerging aromatherapy studies for emotional and cognitive post-menopausal health are promising as a safe, gentle, effective and pleasant option, without the side-effects of multiple medications that create greater risks in this population. Polypharmacy, taking multiple medications from various providers, is an all-too-familiar scenario which brings increased risks of confusion and unpleasant side-effects. Offering alternatives for anxiety, aches and pains and sleep is an ideal starting point to introduce aromatherapy, since medications for these conditions often are taken or increased as needed, rather than regularly scheduled. The combination of medications and external essential oils provides a therapeutic synergy to reduce over-medicating, negative secondary effects and costs, and thus to improve quality of life. The various aromatherapy scents can evoke memories, enhance appetite, ease anxiety, pain, nausea, insomnia and grief, lift spirits, sharpen focus and serve as a valuable therapeutic tool.

Research studies

- Babakhanian *et al.* (2018) A systematic review and meta-analysis of the effect of aromatherapy on the treatment of psychological symptoms in post-menopausal and elderly women.

- Her and Cho (2021), a meta-analysis and systematic review of 30 studies of aromatherapy and sleep quality of adults and elderly, highlighted the following key points:

- Lavender was the essential oil in 26 of the 30 studies.

- Aromatherapy had a positive statistically significant effect on sleep.

- Massage was most effective for sleep with elderly and inpatients.

- Inhalation is effective and methods of inhalation vary from direct on cotton pad to indirect diffuser.

- Frequency and duration of treatments may also be factors to be considered, particularly in residential settings.

- Scuteri *et al.* (2019) studied the neuropsychiatric effects of bergamot essential oil with pain in dementia patients and identified the following:

  - Agitation, irritability, anxiety, aggression and depression can be eased with aromatherapy to improve quality of life.

  - Pain, difficult to communicate and thus undertreated in dementia patients, exhibits as agitation and anxiety.

  - Bergamot in human and animal studies affects neurotransmitter pathways, leading to anxiolytic calming effects and positive behavioral changes.

  - Pain due to inflammation and neuropathic factors was reduced with bergamot, in animal studies as well as human inhalation studies.

- Ballard *et al.* (2002) demonstrated that massage with melissa (lemon balm) reduced agitation scores in dementia patients without side-effects.

Post-menopause–older adult tips

In my experience, older adults often prefer fewer medications and resort to home remedies. Reasons for this include economic factors, fear, and having experienced side-effects from previous medications (Siddiqui *et al.* 2014). Aromatherapy use in the care of elderly physical and emotional conditions is very successful.

Quick reference table: Aromatherapy for post-menopause

Condition	Essential oils	Methods
Anxiety	Lavender, mandarin, rose	Inhalation on cotton pad
Pain	Lavender, bergamot, rosemary, sweet marjoram, Roman chamomile	Dilute in unscented lotion and massage generously on and around area of discomfort
Depression	Lavender, rose	Inhalation 10–30 minutes
Appetite stimulant	Mandarin, bergamot, sweet orange	Cotton ball with oils in medicine cup on meal tray, diffuser
Sleep	Lavender, sweet marjoram	Hand, arm or shoulder massage, cotton pad on gown or bedside diffuser
Sharpen focus	Rosemary, lemon, mint	Cotton pad attached to clothing, diffuser
Agitation	Bergamot, melissa, lavender	Cotton pad attached to clothing, diffuser

Grief and loss

According to Dugas and Slane (2022), it is estimated by the American College of Obstetricians
and Gynecologists (ACOG) that as many as 26
percent, more than one in four, pregnancies end
in miscarriage. As many as 5 percent of women
experience two or more miscarriages, with ensuing feelings of loss and grief. The CDC estimate
for rate of infertility, defined as inability to con-

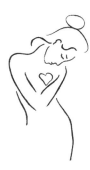

ceive after one year of unprotected intercourse, is 19 percent,
nearly one in five women (CDC 2023). Regardless of identified
male or female fertility issues, women often experience feelings
of guilt, inadequacy, lack of wholeness, grief and/or depression.

For many women, the grief from pregnancy loss, particularly multiple losses, leaves an unfilled space, a gap, a forever
longing, and support from other women with similar losses
provides comfort, connectedness and companionship. Losing
a child at any age is most mothers' worst nightmare, and is
frequently an unrelenting loss that sends them and their family
into unchartered and fractured territory. In-person and online
loss support groups provide necessary understanding and are a
tonic for healing. In many of these groups, facilitators introduce
and utilize aromatherapy for anxiety and depression and to ease
the grief and sadness.

Individual and/or group grief therapy, sometimes long-
term, provide much-needed support and a "port in the storm"
to carry on, navigate guilt, fear, anger and sadness, and function
as well as possible. The experience of aromatherapy easing raw
emotions in safe spaces offers a tool for much-needed self-care

at home. The scent memory of an emotional connection made in therapy is powerful and valuable to access in daily life.

Abortion rates are difficult to obtain. Pew Research (2023) suggests between 600,000 and 900,000 abortions took place in 2019–2020. According to the CDC (2022c), "In 2020, 620,327 legal induced abortions were reported…similar to previous years, in 2020, women in their twenties accounted for more than half of abortions (57.2%). Nearly all abortions in 2020 took place early in gestation: 93.1% of abortions were performed at ≤13 weeks' gestation." Depending on circumstances, which could include ineffective birth control, lack of male or familial support, incest or rape, abortion can lead to fear of exposure, guilt, forbidden grief, loss, sadness, shame and regret that, for some women, can last a lifetime.

Fear of exposure, guilt or shame prevents many women from revealing abortion experiences to anyone. Nurses, midwives and therapists often share intimate communication with women, and this is an important and treasured aspect of our role. We have opportunities to educate, comfort and weave in information about healing modalities such as aromatherapy for shame, loss and guilt, and to offer support and share with them that experiences don't just evaporate; even if they are unvoiced, they can chip away at the woman's mental and emotional health. Regardless of their past, healing is available to all.

In many women, grief from the death of a spouse, divorce or infidelity creates a change in identity, emotional and/or financial security, comfort and companionship.

Feelings of grief or loss for some women reflect nagging missed opportunities, unfulfilled dreams, academic, professional, athletic, artistic or unrealized life adventures hijacked by relationships, unexpected pregnancies, familial obligations and financial constraints. Cumulative loss chips away at a woman's sense of self and may lead to anxiety, depression, self-harm, eating disorders and, in worst-case scenarios, serious mental health conditions.

Self-care with aromatherapy is a valuable tool for the emotional angst and upheaval resulting from any loss. Filling the space with appealing and comforting sensory experiences using therapeutic aromatherapy eases the myriad of fears, pain and anxiety.

In addition, not all loss is negative, albeit a change, and aromatherapy can welcome the renewal, the end of a negative relationship and reconnecting to oneself.

Quick reference table: Grief and loss

Condition	Essential oil	Methods
Grief, loss, anxiety	Rose	Inhalation on cotton pad or personal inhaler. Dilute in jojoba or lotion and apply to wrists and/or chest
Spiritual grief and loss, fear, shock, hyperventilation/ panic	Frankincense	Inhalation on cotton pad or personal inhaler. Spritzer with rose and mandarin or peppermint
Anxiety, insomnia	Lavender	Inhalation on cotton pad or personal inhaler, bath, linen and room spritzer
Sadness and loss	Mandarin	Spritzer with frankincense and rose
Depression, seasonal affective disorder (SAD) intensifying grief, difficult to move on	Bergamot	Room diffuser, spritzer, iinhalation on cotton pad

Condition	Essential oil	Methods
Grief, low energy, congestion from crying, refresh	Peppermint	Inhalation alone or spritzer with frankincense and rose
Need to move forward, new life, renewal, refresh	Yuzu	Diffuser, bath, inhalation
Strength to carry on	Jasmine	Dilute in jojoba, rub on wrists and neck for a therapeutic perfume

Having a professional trusted therapist to process internal thoughts, feelings and behaviors is a gift to oneself for a satisfying, productive life. Mental health therapists can be social workers, nurse therapists, psychologists and counselors with various age and treatment specialties, so referrals from physicians, nurse practitioners or trusted friends are important in finding a good fit. Universities generally have mental health therapists at low to no cost to students, which are so valuable at this critical time in older teen and young adult lives.

Anger/rage and chronic conditions

Historically, females' relationships with their feelings and suppression of the natural emotion of anger, in many cases rage, present as anxiety, depression, physical pain and unhealthy internal and external communication. In many cultures anger is considered a male emotion and "unladylike" to experience or express. The feelings are real, anger is a natural human emotion and without an outlet, the confusing mixed message internally intensifies, wreaking havoc on physical and mental health.

It has been said that "depression is anger turned inward," and with the current rates of depression one could surmise that there's a great deal of unexpressed anger lurking inside of many females. Lifetimes of hearing "smile and look pretty," "nice girls don't raise their voices," "you're just an angry feminist," against a backdrop of daily accounts of physical and sexual abuse, infidelities, clergy and coach abuse of our children, incest and rape, reproductive privacy and rights stripped away, without any male responsibility for unexpected pregnancies take their toll.

Many young girls and women have lacked female role models that demonstrate healthy ways of processing anger. The absence of female dialogue and education regarding the acceptability of "feeling angry," a normal and justified emotion, often leads to them suppressing this emotion, which can over time result in mental and physical health conditions.

According to recent studies specifically on cardiac risk factors, anger, depression and stress in women (Chida and Steptoe 2009; Schmidt *et al.* 2018), there is a complex relationship between anger and higher rates of cardiovascular events and conditions in women, and it is important to acknowledge and heighten awareness of this. According to Smeijers *et al.* (2017), cardiovascular system events are potentiated in the first two hours following outbursts of anger, with a fivefold increase in heart attack incidence and threefold increase in stroke risk, with the risk increasing with repeated outbursts.

Anger management and stress reduction techniques are recommended to reduce physical and mental health risk factors, and aromatherapy offers therapeutic options, shared throughout this guidebook, to ease anger, depression, anxiety and stress.

The therapeutic benefit of aromatherapy with anger is protective self-care, smoothing the rough edges, instilling strength and fortitude to manage the miserable feelings, and clarity of thought for a way forward without self-destruction. Unresolved anger potentiates physical and emotional distress, intensifying PMS, menstrual discomforts, depression, anxiety, pain and heart health.

Quick reference table: Anger and rage

Condition	Essential oil	Methods
Anger, rage, irritability	Ylang-ylang	Inhalation
Anxiety, depression, loss of love	Rose	Inhalation
Anxiety, insomnia	Lavender	Inhalation, linen spray
Insecurity, lack of confidence	Jasmine	Inhalation on a cotton pad or personal inhaler, dilute in jojoba oil and apply to wrists
Exhaustion, worsening PMS or menopausal symptoms	Geranium	Inhalation, if appealing. Dilute in lotion and massage over lower abdomen, wrists and or/ adrenal area twice daily during PMS or menopausal worsening
Confusion, focus issues	Rosemary	Inhalation on cotton pad or personal inhaler
Low energy, sluggish	Lemon	Inhalation or spritzer with rosemary or jasmine or geranium or lavender

Women and scent: Attraction and love

As the stories and legends go, Cleopatra draped her sails with roses/rosewater to seduce Mark Anthony; Mary Magdalene massaged Jesus' feet with precious spikenard; the coronation anointing of Queen Elizabeth II and kings and queens before her was a blend of rose, cinnamon, jasmine, musk, benzoin, civet, orange flower and ambergris in sesame and olive oil. History demonstrates the power, seduction and beauty of women and scent. Aromatics envelop and complete our package of beauty and self-care as well as extending far beyond us to others' memories of us. Many can remember the scents of their mothers, friends or lovers long after they're gone from our lives. Opening these spaces in others with aromatherapy enters the unseen "healing spaces" to lessen suffering and grief, and improve mental health.

Women's menstrual cycle, hormones, scent and emotions

According to Fung *et al.* (2021), "The olfactory system is unique among the sensory systems for having direct anatomical and functional links with the limbic system, thus olfactory stimuli have a strong effect on mood."

Women's sense of smell is more sensitive than that of males, responding well to aromatherapy during hormonal and emotional upheaval. According to multiple studies (Bogdan *et al.* 2021; Graham *et al.* 2003; Matsumoto *et al.* 2016; Watanabe *et al.* 2002), changing hormone levels throughout the menstrual cycle affect the intensity and appeal of various scents. In the beginning of your cycle, just after the end of menses, estrogen levels are low and the sense of smell is at its lowest; as the levels rise daily, so does the discrimination and/or appreciation of various scents. As estrogen levels rise mid-cycle, women experience scents more acutely, and post-ovulation, with rises in progesterone, the sense of taste increases, perhaps to prepare for fueling a pregnancy. In the premenstrual week, estrogen decreases, many women become irritable and annoyed, and many scents can be overpowering, even those enjoyed earlier in the cycle. As estrogen drops, it makes you more sensitive to sensory input of all kinds. Matsumoto *et al.*'s (2013) study indicated that women inhaling lavender for 10 minutes experienced significantly reduced irritability and anger and improved overall mood. In practice, we've experienced a similar positive premenstrual response with twice-daily inhalations and diluted skin applications to the wrists and lower abdomen with a blend of equal parts geranium, ylang-ylang and clary sage essential oils for 7–10 days prior to menses.

Women with anosmia, the inability to smell, have higher rates of depression than women with the ability to smell (Hur *et al.* 2018). Our sense of smell is so vital to the pleasures of cooking, tasting, gardening, environmental enhancement and sensing danger that if it is compromised, it negatively affects our quality of life. Women with amenorrhea, the lack of menstrual periods, also experience greater rates of depression, thus indicating on many levels the importance of our senses for optimal biological and psychological functioning.

As we decorate the outside of our homes to gift our neighbors, so we spritz our bodies with beautiful scents we only smell upon application. The US fragrance industry revenues for 2022 are $8.15bn—clear testimony to the desirability and popularity of scented products for making us feel and smell better and attracting others.

Cultural considerations

Culturally, scented plants indigenous to or abundant in one's homeland, laced with memories, offer uplifting therapeutic options for depression and anxiety. In practice, the addition of a cultural scent assessment opens a magical space for treatment success. Ask questions such as "What grows in the area you grew up or your favorite vacation area?," "What scents do you remember that were pleasant to you and/or remind you of a loved one?" or, equally, "Do any scents carry unpleasant memories for you?" In times of depression or grief, a familiar scent from a happier time has the potential to lift spirits and transport a person to a time when life was more pleasant for them. I've found this very effective with postpartum depression, menopause and elderly loneliness, grief and depression.

The following are examples that may be beneficial or, depending on circumstances, could be triggers of past traumas:

- Rose: Often used in cooking, confectionary, bath and skin products in Middle Eastern countries.

- Pine, juniper and sage: Used ceremonially, spiritually and medicinally by Native Americans.

- Citrus: Widely grown, scents the air and consumed in warm, sunny regions.

- Ylang-ylang: South American and Pacific island natives use as perfumery and in celebrations.

- Jasmine: Indian celebrations, weddings and perfumery; tea for winter depression.

- Lavender: France, European linens, sleep and skincare, sachets, honey, potpourri, confectionery, gardens and farms.

- Chamomile: Mexican healing remedy as a tea for multiple infirmities.

- Rosemary: Mediterranean "remembrance," gardens, culinary.

- Peppermint: North American Christmas holiday candy canes, teas and digestive support.

- Sandalwood: Indian base of many aromatics, traditions and ceremonies.

- Cinnamon: Sri Lanka, West Indies, Mexico, Americas— old and most familiar culinary spice.

This is not an exhaustive list. In practice with depression, grief, homesickness, anxiety and sadness, scent memories of a far-away home, people or holidays can be quickly uplifting.

Evidence-based mental health essential oil list

Most studies measure stress, anxiety and depression, which are components of every single mental health condition. In other words, an individual in a manic or psychotic state, even if not diagnosed with general anxiety disorder, is experiencing anxiety and can be helped with aromatherapy for anxiety.

Lavender *(lavandula angustifolia)*

Lavender is the most studied essential oil for multiple conditions, with overwhelmingly statistically positive responses. Kim *et al.'s* (2021) systematic review and meta-analysis of 21 lavender studies indicated favorable reductions of anxiety, and decreased heart rate, systolic blood pressure, cortisol (the stress hormone) and CgA (an indicator of anxiety/depression) with inhalation of lavender in multiple settings. Abdelhakim *et al.'s* (2020) meta-analysis and systematic review of nine aromatherapy and cardiac surgery randomized control trials (RCTs), predominantly using lavender by inhalation, showed a decrease in anxiety, pain and heart rate.

The chemical constituents in high percentage, linalool and linalyl acetate, contribute to the calming and sedative therapeutic properties. However, at times, a paradoxical reaction has been noted with lavender in children where lavender stimulates rather than calms, which is probably due to the immature GABA system in the younger brain. As a result of this potential, it is best to use 1% in children, which is often quite effective and pleasant for the child. Inhalations, massage or baths are the most common methods. Asthmatics and those with seasonal allergies can have a negative allergic-type respiratory response *so always check with them and respect the potential regardless of brand, especially with a history of asthma.* In practice, I have witnessed this reaction on several occasions.

Silexan 1 is a patented active substance with an essential oil produced from *lavandula angustifolia* flowers by steam distillation. Silexan is formulated in a soft gelatin capsule containing 80 mg of lavender oil, and it has been authorized in Germany as a medicinal product for the treatment of states of restlessness related to anxious mood. In a double-blind, placebo-controlled, randomized clinical trial, silexan showed superiority over placebo in 221 adults suffering from subsyndromal anxiety disorder (Kasper *et al.* 2010). Similarly, 80 mg of silexan administered for six weeks was shown to be as effective as 0.5 mg of lorazepam in 77 patients suffering from generalized anxiety disorder (Woelk and Schlafke 2010). Additionally, a better tolerability of silexan compared to paroxetine has been confirmed in a trial including 539 generalized anxiety disorder patients (Kasper *et al.* 2014). Moreover, the effectiveness of silexan has been demonstrated in patients with neurasthenia, post-traumatic stress disorder, and somatization disorder regarding the efficiency of sleep and mood improvement (Uehleke *et al.* 2012).

Rose *(rosa damascena)*

Multiple women's health studies involving rose have had statistically positive findings for anxiety, postpartum and general depression. Known as the "queen of oils," its range of emotional and physical therapeutic properties for adult women with PMS, infertility, labor, postpartum depression, menopause and grief is due to nearly 300 chemical constituents at interplay throughout the hypothalamic-pituitary-axis (HPA), endocrine and neurological, memory and cultural pathways. It is expensive, but well worth the investment. Treatments are effective with 1–2% inhalation or hand or shoulder massage. Mohebitabar *et al.*'s (2017) review of 13 clinical studies with rose oil demonstrated positive anti-anxiety, antidepressant and analgesic findings by inhalation or massage. Burns *et al*'s (2000) eight-year intrapartum study rated rose as most effective for anxiety in labor. Multiple dysmenorrhea studies have shown that rose alone or in a blend decreased menstrual pain and anxiety (Han *et al.* 2017; Marzouk *et al.* 2013; Sadeghi *et al.* 2014; Uysal *et al.* 2016*)*. Menopausal studies with rose alone or in blend showed positively decreased anxiety and depression and noted increased salivary estrogen level. Cultural and memory assessments are important with rose due to the aromatic association with joyful and traumatic life events, which can be positive or negative emotional triggers. This is a valuable tool in mental health aromatherapy.

Sweet orange *(citrus sinensis)*

In procedural, dental and clinical waiting room studies, sweet orange demonstrates positive responses, decreasing anxiety and providing an uplifting cheerful environment. In a diffuser or by direct inhalation on a cotton pad, it is a simple and familiar cheerful scent that can reduce anxiety and fear, particularly in children and the elderly. In labor (Rashidi *et al.* 2013) and postpartum (Asazawa *et al.* 2017) studies with sweet orange by inhalation or massage significantly decreased anxiety.

Neroli *(citrus aurantium)*

In cardiac procedures, labor, colonoscopy, pediatric emergency room and intensive care units (ICU), anxiety decreased and vital signs improved with inhalations, massage and/or diffusers with neroli (Cho *et al.* 2013; Holm and Fitzmaurice 2008; Hu *et al.* 2010; Moslemi *et al.* 2019; Scandurra *et al.* 2022). Although it's an expensive oil, only 1–2 drops are needed per treatment and in higher acuity areas with accompanying anxiety, it's very effective. Mannucci *et al.*'s (2018) comparison of nine anxiety studies of sweet orange and neroli demonstrated neroli as a more effective anxiolytic than sweet orange.

Bergamot *(citrus bergamia)*

A mental health center waiting room study of 50 women (Han *et al.* 2017) with diffusion of bergamot for 15 minutes showed significantly improved positive feelings in an anxiety producing environment. A dementia study (Scuteri *et al.* 2019) with bergamot showed anxiolytic effects without the sedation side effects of benzodiazepines, thus increasing safety. A post-partum depression center study (Chen *et al.* 2022) of 60 women diffused bergamot in an atomizer diffuser versus water for 15 minutes each afternoon for four weeks. Data indicated women in the aromatherapy group had significantly lower depressive mood scores than those in the control water group at two and four weeks.

Roman chamomile *(chamaemelum nobile)*

Roman chamomile is a well-known popular remedy for sleep and anxiety. Burns *et al.*'s (2000, 2007) intrapartum studies found that of 6–10 essential oils, Roman chamomile was one of two oils most helpful for labor pain. (The other was clary sage.)

Frankincense (boswellia carterii)

Terminal hospice patients received aromatherapy massages on each hand for five minutes for seven consecutive days using a blend of bergamot, lavender and frankincense with significant decreased depression and pain than the control group (Chang 2008).

Other essential oils beneficial to mental health

- Lemon (*citrus limon*)

- Mandarin (*citrus reticulata*)

- Jasmine (*jasminum officinale*)

- Rosemary (*rosmarinus officinalis*)

- Ylang-ylang (*cananga odorata*)

- Geranium (*pelargonium graveolens*)

- Clary sage (*salvia sclarea*)

- Melissa (*melissa officinalis*)

- Yuzu (*citrus junos*)

- Petitgrain (*citrus bigaradia*)

- Sandalwood (*santalum album*)

- Peppermint (*mentha piperita*)

- Sweet marjoram (*origanum majorana*)

Quick reference table: Evidence-based essential oils for anxiety and/or depression

Conditions	Essential oil	Methods
Anxiety with all conditions, depression	Lavender	Inhalation, spray, diffuser, massage, bath
Anxiety, depression, grief	Rose	Inhalation, spray, massage, bath
Anxiety, depression	Sweet orange	Inhalation, spray, diffuser
Anxiety, panic	Neroli	Inhalation, spray, massage
Anxiety, depression	Bergamot	Inhalation, spray, diffuser, massage
Anxiety, depression	Roman chamomile	Inhalation, massage
Panic, anxiety, hyperventilation, grief *Avoid with psychotic clients*	Frankincense	Inhalation, spray
Anxiety, depression	Lemon	Inhalation, spray, diffuser, massage
Anxiety, depression	Mandarin	Inhalation, spray, diffuser
Anxiety, depression	Jasmine	Inhalation, spray, massage, diffuser
Anxiety, depression, mental focus	Rosemary	Inhalation, spray, diffuser
Anxiety, irritability	Ylang-ylang	Inhalation, spray, diffuser, massage, bath
Anxiety, PMS	Geranium	Inhalation, massage
Anxiety, depression, menses, labor, PMS, menopause	Clary sage	Inhalation, massage

Anxiety, depression	Melissa (lemon balm)	Inhalation, spray, diffuser
Anxiety, depression	Yuzu	Inhalation, spray, diffuser, baths
Anxiety, depression	Petitgrain	Inhalation, spray, diffuser
Anxiety	Sandalwood	Inhalation, massage, spray
Depression	Peppermint	Inhalation, diffuser, spray *Avoid near cardiac patients, babies and young children*
Anxiety	Sweet marjoram	Massage/skin application

CHAPTER 5

The Healing Space

A sacred space within us, where music enlivens, uplifts and touches our souls, where we escape into a work of art, forgetting our pain and grief, where a wafting scent evokes the memory of a lover or security of the kitchen of our childhood, stimulating pleasant faraway sensations, our senses hold a rich pathway to our emotions and our healing. At this time, we lack the tools to measure most of the effects of our senses, but we are keenly aware of how we feel when exposed to sensory stimuli that delight us. I'll take a leap to name this "The Healing Space," where through our senses we're able to access a purer, more divine part of ourselves.

Aromatherapy invokes the sense of smell via our olfactory system and stimulates pathways to our memories, emotions and hormones. Scientific studies, the aromatherapy evidence base, demonstrate the lowering and raising of our heart rate, blood pressure, respiration, and neurotransmitter, adrenal, pituitary and stress hormone levels from inhalation or massage/ skin application with essential oils. The subjective response, "how the scent made me feel," and the objective scientific, measurable responses of vital signs and blood levels pre/post-aromatherapy treatments make aromatherapy a valuable tool for therapists. Each client or patient presents with a tapestry of scent memories, positive and negative, cultural programming related to the symbolism of scent and to culinary rituals, traditions, religious and sacred beliefs, ceremony, romance, pleasure and self-care. For example, the scent of rose is abundant in Middle Eastern culture in everyday food, confections, celebrations and festivals, all reminiscent of ordinary and joyful events, and in the US the strong scent of rose is often associated with funerals, a sad or traumatic event. Including the client in the selection of a therapeutic oil by offering 2–5 choices and asking if there are any scents that they find pleasant or even unappealing is a most effective and personal approach. The effect is quite immediate; with a depressed individual, a smile appears or eyes brighten when they inhale a scent pleasant to them, and with an anxious person, they breathe more easily, tension eases and they experience a welcome calming effect. On multiple occasions in my practice, when treating depression clinically, a client would have a completely flat affect with a number of oils known for their antidepressant properties, then noticeably brighten smelling mandarin. There is a space, a healing space, within us all which is accessible through the combination of a pleasant scent, surfacing a long-buried memory of a happier time, a shift in our feelgood chemicals and/or appreciation of a gentle gift of aroma shared between therapist and client.

CHAPTER 6

Aromatherapy to Support Emotional Health in Women's Cardiology and Breast Cancer

Integrative Therapy

Anxiety and depression coexist with multiple medical conditions, increasing their progression and risk factors. If emotions are ignored, preventable and treatable conditions worsen and a minor scenario develops into a serious, potentially life-threatening one. In multiple studies, aromatherapy interventions for anxiety, fear and depression have demonstrated significant positive responses, improving stress hormone levels and vital signs, thus lessening risks and leading to improved outcomes.

Breast cancer

Breast cancer, the most common malignancy in women worldwide, is many women's most feared condition. It draws to mind images of hair loss from chemotherapy and surgical removal of breasts, thus altering the female body and emotionally changing a woman's sense of self, femininity, attractiveness and desirability as well as fears of mortality. This is an experience laced not only with concerns for themselves, but also fears for their children's futures and family wellbeing.

Aromatherapy eases symptoms of nausea and anxiety during treatment as well as enhancing pleasant scents for the myriad of emotional and spiritual upheavals that can occur during and at the end of treatments. In our weekly two-hour afternoon breast cancer support group, a diffuser welcomed the women with an uplifting and anti-nausea blend of peppermint, rosemary and sweet orange. After two years together, none of the active treatment clients had become nauseated or fallen asleep during group, a common occurrence during acute treatment, and all appreciated the blend. At one point, to evaluate aromatherapy as a tool to reduce anxiety, all of the clients consented to evaluate their anxiety and their comfort communicating in group about topics such as intimacy and fear of death at the beginning and end of the group session. They rated anxiety and willingness to communicate difficult topics pre- and post- on a Likert 0–10 scale and we found that a blend of mandarin and lavender successfully calmed anxieties and uplifted the clients emotionally, and an increase in spontaneous laughter-filled conversation occurred: all positive experiences. Guided imagery with a choice of mandarin or lavender on a cotton pad to take home ended the sessions, with regular feedback of lessened anxiety and stress and increased optimism, which continued throughout the week.

A few studies measuring a variety of complementary therapies for breast cancer have shown positive results with aromatherapy (Deng *et al.* 2022; Imanishi *et al.* 2009; Tola *et al.* 2021).

Cardiology

Cardiovascular events and procedures, with their life-threatening risks and fears, are frequently accompanied by anxiety and, if serious or prolonged, depression. Pre-menopausal women, who have cardioprotective estrogen, have fewer heart attacks, strokes and overall cardiac events than men. The rates after menopause are very similar. Depression, anxiety and myocardial infarction (MI) (heart attacks) are a dangerous combination and combined can lead to further heart attacks. Anxiety increases cortisol, a stress hormone, causing heart rate, respiration and blood pressure to increase, which has a potential effect on risk factors and recurrence.

Women's heart health has gained significant attention in the past 20 years, possibly due to increased numbers of female physicians, scientists and clinical researchers providing a voice at the table and highlighting gender differences in cardiology. Marketing women's heart health around Valentine's Day and fashionable red clothing has enhanced societal awareness of gender differences and risk factors. Historically, the majority of studies in cardiology were conducted on males, with medications and treatments adjusted for females by weight. In multiple studies, aromatherapy with various essential oils reduced levels of the stress hormone cortisol, which is critically important during a crisis, trauma, loss or cardiac events.

According to Prasad (2007), "Takotsubo cardiomyopathy," commonly known as "broken heart syndrome," is a condition that most often occurs in post-menopausal women aged 58–75 after a traumatic breakup, accident or sudden intense trauma or grief. The symptoms are similar to a heart attack. The precise cause isn't known, but experts think that surging stress hormones (i.e. cortisol, adrenaline) essentially "stun" the heart, triggering changes in heart muscle cells or coronary blood vessels (or both) that prevent the left ventricle from contracting effectively. If treated immediately, most people recover rapidly with no long-term heart damage. Aromatherapy can help by lowering cortisol to decrease added stress on the heart.

The first 48 hours after a myocardial infarction is the most unstable and vulnerable time to experience a second, often more serious cardiac event; however, higher risk factors remain for 90 days up to five years. In addition to initial life-saving procedures, rest and medications, lifestyle changes are prescribed to include therapeutic modalities for stress reduction and mental health. Depression incidence is higher overall in women and often increases following a heart attack, intensifying the risk factors for cardiac events and necessitating therapeutic modalities such as aromatherapy to ease depression and reduce risks. Cardiology studies (Mattina *et al.* 2019; Nair *et al.* 2021; Peters *et al.* 2021) confirm the complex relationship between depression and heart health in women. Multiple aromatherapy studies highlight significant positive cardiovascular and mental health results.

Aromatherapy for anxiety reduction in cardiology settings

A sampling of cardiology aromatherapy studies demonstrates significant positive results decreasing anxiety and stress and maintaining hemodynamic balance with simple inhalations of either rose, lavender, melissa, geranium, neroli or roman chamomile. In frightening, potentially life-threatening situations, aromatherapy provides a pleasant, painless and effective therapeutic option to improve the experience for both the patient and the caregiver.

Aromatherapy for anxiety reduction in clinical settings

- Intensive care unit intubation: Inhalations for 30 minutes of neroli or lavender.

- Intensive care unit: Inhalations of lavender, Roman chamomile and neroli.

- Myocardial infarction: Inhalations of lavender twice daily for two days.

- Acute myocardial infarction: Rose inhalations three times daily for three days decreased pain intensity and anxiety.

- Coronary ER: Inhalations of melissa.

- Intravenous (IV) stick: Inhalations of lavender.

- Surgical and procedural anxiety: Inhalations of lavender, sweet orange or rose.

- Intrauterine device placement: Inhalations of lavender.

- Epidural placement: Inhalations of lavender or rose.

- Breast surgery: Inhalations of lavender.

- Premenstrual syndrome (PMS): Ylang-ylang, clary sage, geranium, rose lotion or inhalation of all blended or any singly.

- Labor: Inhalations or massage with lavender, rose.

- Postpartum: Rose, lavender and jasmine lotion, inhalations of mandarin, rose, or frankincense if panicky.

- Menopause: Geranium, rose, ylang-ylang, clary sage.

CHAPTER 7

Helping Women Have Better Mental Health

Prescription medications have improved many lives and altered the need for institutional care of many with serious mental health disorders such as schizophrenia, bipolar manic depressive conditions and severe depression, as more individuals on these medications are able to function in society.

In mental health, medication compliance, taking medication as prescribed, is often a strong factor in treatment success. The range of noncompliance rates found in different studies, worse with serious psychiatric conditions, is 24–90% (Semahegn *et al.* 2020). Many prefer to avoid medications for anxiety and mild-to-moderate depression, while others struggle with compliance, that is, staying on their medications. The reasons for avoiding medications are varied and include fears of addiction with anti-anxiety medications, unpleasant side-effects, having to wait two to four weeks for improvements with antidepressants, potential for worsening of symptoms and, for younger adults, a higher risk of suicide with certain antidepressants; hence the black box warning on the side of these bottles.

Medical evaluations are necessary to rule out potential underlying conditions that can exacerbate and intensify emotions. Women's hormonal cycles can worsen symptoms of anxiety and depression every month for some, after childbirth for many and in perimenopause and menopause for others. Affirming that all systems are in balance provides assurance that emotional states are not caused by masked physical conditions.

Therapeutic levels of medications are important for adequate treatment of conditions. Guidance on medications and dosages from physicians and pharmacists offers the most qualified expertise. It's very important that any weaning off or discontinuing of psychiatric medications be done with medical supervision as symptoms can worsen if stopped abruptly.

Regardless of diagnosis and/or severity of illness, aromatherapy used externally can be incorporated into a self-care regimen. If on medications, internal use of essential oils can compete with the medication at the receptor site, potentiating or weakening the medication, so it is best to avoid this method.

Aromatherapy and women's mental health basics

Aromatherapy, for the purpose of this book, refers to both *aroma*: the scent of the essential oils derived from an aromatic plant, and *therapy*: the use of the aromatic essential oils for measurable therapeutic purposes.

There are many "gurus" in this field as well as massive essential oil sales companies with extensive marketing campaigns readily available and enthusiastic to supply their oils, blends and brands, often without adequate education or qualifications for clinical recommendations. For this book, we'll focus on the clinical: the actual therapeutic experience of nurses, therapists, midwives and patients in clinical settings, as well as the available published aromatherapy studies: the evidence base.

In the UK, nursing and midwifery hospital aromatherapy programs started in the 1980s as a non-pharmacological complementary therapy to ease patients' anxiety, pain and nausea. In every clinical program to date, anxiety is the most common patient complaint and has been successfully decreased in thousands of treatments worldwide. Results from large older clinical oncology and midwifery studies (Burns *et al.* 2000; Wilkenson *et al.* 2007) have been replicated in multiple recent studies. In other words, ample clinical data spanning 30 years exists to indicate aromatherapy is an effective and safe option in the toolkit for mental health.

Aromatherapy for stress management has long been accepted as an enjoyable spa-like therapy to create a pleasant, calm environment. This can be done in your office, home or car and, though aromatherapy is a complementary, not alternative, therapy or a cure for mental illness, in this book we will explore results of hundreds of studies—the evidence base for improving anxiety, depression, fear and panic disorders.

The increasingly complex roles women navigate and how far we stretch ourselves are all taking a toll on our mental and emotional health. Images of the perfect physical appearance, impressive career, relationships, marriage, mothering, caring for children and parents, beautiful home, fashionable clothing, culinary skills, athletic performance and so much more, in some measure weigh heavily on our minds, how we feel emotionally, and daily self-judging, the continuous loop on replay. Women face challenges with weight and body image, fertility issues, beauty defined by culture, history of physical or sexual abuse, abortion, single motherhood, financial challenges, grief, loss, not fitting into others' molds and unfulfilled dreams. There are endless realities chipping away at the fibers of the quality of many women's lives and wellbeing.

Women's bodies cycle through an intricate balance of hormonal levels that affect both our emotional and physical feelings and sensations. Our inherited genetics and our life experiences can dramatically alter the severity of our monthly symptoms and understanding the basics of how this all functions can be both enlightening and healing. Women's intuition that "something just isn't right" is very real and a distinct aspect of our knowing, our unique intelligence. Collective female wisdom, passed from one female to another, often learned at the kitchen table of our childhood, sparks, enriches and guides that intelligence. It is a powerful tool and too often ignored as an aspect of our mind–body intelligence.

CHAPTER 8

Methods and Safety

Methods

The method used for aromatherapy is critical: *more is not better* and evidence-based methods enhance the therapeutic effect.

In mental health care, direct inhalation or indirect use via diffuser or spritzer will be the optimal methods the majority of time; they're fast-acting, pleasant, and offer quick reduction of symptoms and/or de-escalation of a more serious situation. Internal use is not recommended; it lacks evidence base and potentially interferes with medication receptors, making them less effective or potentiating them in some cases. Anecdotally, nurses on mental health units certified in clinical aromatherapy have reported a 30 percent lower seclude and restrain monthly rate when a diffuser with lavender was used with permission daily for 30 days. As a group therapy facilitator for three years, I found our patients reported decreased anxiety and enhanced willingness to approach difficult topics when diffusing mandarin and lavender. Frankincense, although very relaxing in normal situations where it can reduce anxiety, panic or grief, has a unique property of increasing lability in psychiatric patients with a history of thought disorders, and I have personally witnessed the unwelcome chaos with the oil in a group setting. Although not dangerous, the experience was unpleasant for those affected. In a two-year cancer support group of patients in active treatment, peppermint, sweet orange and rosemary were diffused 30 minutes prior to the start of the group. There was no incidence of sleeping or becoming nauseated during the two-hour afternoon group. At the end of group, a guided imagery exercise with individual inhalations of mandarin or lavender anchored the scent with a relaxing exercise they continued at home with positive results.

Massages or baths are often unavailable or inappropriate in mental health facilities, although both are excellent for stress reduction.

The importance of ongoing aromatherapy self-care can be demonstrated in the practitioner's office by inhaling two or three oils to determine personal preference or, with permission, using an office diffuser or spray just before the session. Many practitioners spray before and after sessions for antiseptic and energetic self-care.

"Caring for the caregiver" is the most important aspect of clinical aromatherapy. By caring for ourselves, we're better equipped to care for others. Mental health for all!

The methods used in women's mental health are all external:

- Inhalation: Direct: 1–3 drops on cotton pad or personal inhaler; indirect: with diffuser.
  The quickest and most effective route for anxiety, panic, fear, nausea.

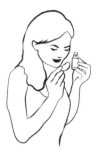

● Skin application/massage: Dilute 1–5 drops essential oils for healthy non-pregnant adults in 5 ml unscented lotion or carrier oil (e.g., grapeseed, jojoba, fractionated coconut oil).

Best route for any physical pain and discomfort.

If the patient has recently undergone surgery, avoid suture line until stitches are removed and completely healed.

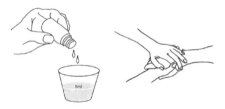

● Baths (whole body, sitz or footbaths): Add 2–8 drops essential oils to carrier oil for dispersion, then add mix to warm bath water.

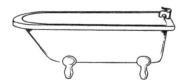

- Spritzer: Add oils (12 gtt/1 oz bottle) to a glass spray bottle, fill with sterile water, shake and spray. Excellent for hot flashes, refreshing for athletes and long days, creating personal space for women around the clinical area.

   For long-term spritzer spray shelf life add dispersant such as perfume alcohol, vodka or solubol.

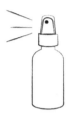

Blending

Mix essential oils together first then add blended drops to lotion or carrier oil before skin application OR on cotton round for inhalation OR to sterile water in spray bottle.

Example: Add lavender 3 drops, lemon 1 drop together, then to make a 1% blend you would add 1 gtt total of this blend to 1 tsp/5 ml of carrier lotion.

- 1 gtt in 5 ml lotion = 1%, 2 gtt in 5 ml lotion = 2%

- To make a 1% blend, add 12 drops total of essential oil to a 2 oz/60 ml bottle of carrier oil, or 2 oz/60ml of lotion… SHAKE WELL

- Always write your blends down.

CHAPTER 9

Mental Health Aromatherapy Evidence Base

The vast majority of human aromatherapy studies have measured mental health conditions, primarily anxiety, depression and/or stress, in multiple clinical specialties ranging from cardiac to university females with menstrual disorders. Generally, the measurements were standardized anxiety and depression tools and subjective pre/post-aromatherapy treatment participant responses. The data overwhelmingly indicates improvement and statistically positive responses with the use of aromatherapy. The practical beauty of the clinical evidence base is the ability to step away from exclusively mental health and inpatient psychiatric units to all specialties of medicine and society at large; anxiety, depression and stress are endemic in modern society. Let's explore the current evidence base for the most prevalent issues.

Anxiety

Anxiety is an emotion which is characterized by an unpleasant state of inner turmoil and includes feelings of dread over anticipated events (Chand and Marwaha 2022). The silent epidemic of anxiety can range from occasional worry and nervousness to full-blown, crippling panic attacks. Benzodiazepines (Xanax, Ativan, Valium) are the most common anti-anxiety medications. They are effective, and best for short-term use as needed with panic disorders; however, they can lead to physical addiction and tolerance and have numerous side-effects impacting daily life. The SSRI (selective serotonin release inhibitor) antidepressants such as Prozac, Zoloft, Celebrex, Paxil and Lexapro are also prescribed for anxiety. They have fewer issues with addiction, but they take weeks of regular use to reduce anxiety so can't be used as an as-needed option, and they are mainly used with chronic anxiety problems that require ongoing treatment. Cognitive behavior therapy (CBT), mindfulness meditation, deep breathing, exercise and yoga are all common treatments and for many, at least initially, a potpourri of therapies is necessary. In this book we'll dive into the evidence base and decades of global clinical practice that reinforce the untapped potential aromatherapy offers for the wide range of anxiety disorders.

Essential oils and anxiety

In nearly 400 published aromatherapy and anxiety studies, the essential oils most often studied with positive results in order of effectiveness are the following:

- *Lavender (*lavandula angustifolia*): "the most often studied essential oil" (Kang *et al.* 2019)

- *Rose (*rosa damascena*)

- Sweet orange (*citrus sinensis*)

- *Neroli (*citrus aurantium*)

- *Frankincense (*boswellia carterii*)

- *Bergamot (*citrus bergamia*)

- *Mandarin (*citrus reticulata*)

- *Roman chamomile (*chamaemelum nobile*)

- *Lemon (*citrus limon*)

- Rosemary (*rosmarinus officinalis*)

- *Geranium (*pelargonium graveolens*)

- *Ylang-ylang (*cananga odorata*)

- *Clary sage (*salvia sclarea*)

- Sweet marjoram (*origanum majorana*)

- *Yuzu (*citrus junos*)

- Melissa (*melissa officinalis*)

* Oils used successfully for anxiety in multiple clinical settings by author

If you're just starting to use essential oils for anxiety personally or in your mental health practice, start simply with lavender, sweet orange or mandarin, lemon, rose and frankincense.

The sensation of anxiety can range from "butterflies in the stomach," a common reaction to new uncomfortable situations, to incapacitating panic attacks in professional or relationship scenarios. According to the World Health Organization (WHO 2022), "In the first year of the COVID-19 pandemic, global prevalence of anxiety and depression increased by a massive 25%." The likelihood is that a 50% increase is probably closer to reality based on increased online therapy offerings, vast shortage of services, incentives for education in mental health fields, and communication with a range of psychological practitioners, all noting increases in their patient population and referrals. In other words, in modern society, there exists an "anxiety epidemic." Rates are always higher in females than males; this is likely due to the ever-shifting hormonal, neurotransmitter and stress levels exacerbating anxiety with the ebbs, flows, interruptions and cessations of the menstrual cycle. Familiarizing oneself with trigger times and situations can guide aromatherapy as well as other self-care options. Inhalation, the quickest and most effective method for anxiety, is simple—either essential oil drops on a cotton pad, tissue or inhaler or, if needed, directly from the bottle. Monthly aromatic massages, if possible, and baths, ideally twice-weekly, are lovely and wonderful when time permits. Herbal and nutritional remedies such as ashwagandha and L-theanine can also offer support. At times, short-term prescribed medication is important for the roughest patches, and that's ok, with the guidance of the person's doctor, nurse practitioner and therapist.

CHAPTER 10

Emerging Science

Neurotransmitters and HPA Systems: The Basics

"How does aromatherapy work?":
Potential mechanisms of action

Neurotransmitters are chemical messengers in our nervous systems that pass signals via neurons. If neurotransmitter levels are too high or too low it can lead to a wide range of mental health issues, most notably anxiety and depression, which are this book's primary foci.

Several recent studies have explored the effects of essential oil inhalation, diffusion and massage on hypothalamic-pituitary axis (HPA) and neurotransmitter levels.[1]

The chemical constituents of the essential oils provide the measurable therapeutic effect. The focus in this book is primarily the sedative/calming and stimulating/uplifting properties. Even with more serious psychotic/thought disorder conditions,

---

1   According to Sheng *et al.* (2021), "The hypothalamic-pituitary-adrenal axis is a complex system of neuroendocrine pathways and feedback loops that function to maintain physiological homeostasis. It mediates the effects of stressors by regulating numerous physiological processes, such as metabolism, immune responses, and the autonomic nervous system."

aromatherapy can reduce anxiety in these terrifying states, thus leading to improved behaviors and favorable outcomes. In inpatient psychiatric settings and support groups, I've witnessed a calming and de-escalation of tense situations with a diffuser or room spray with lavender or mandarin essential oil. Most people experience varying degrees of anxiety in unfamiliar or clinical settings and minimal single oil aromatherapy has been shown to reduce these feelings, leading to a more harmonious and less dangerous environment.

Lavender (*lavandula angustifolia*), the most studied essential oil, is rich with the chemicals linalool and linalyl acetate, which are both major contributors to its well-known relaxing effects. Exploration in several studies of other oils possessing these constituents has demonstrated the same effect, adding to the repertoire of choices for anxiety. Due to seasonal allergies, asthma and scent preference, despite its popularity, lavender is not for everyone, so it is always best to inquire.

Recent studies have measured changes in the stress hormone cortisol, the neurotransmitters GABA and serotonin/5 HTP, and the HPA, as well as objective responses to feelings and quality of life indicators before and after aromatherapy treatments (Fung *et al.* 2021; Lizarraga-Valderrama 2021; Lv *et al.* 2013). Understanding the underlying responses and reactions on a deeper level enhances the potential of aromatherapy as a relevant supportive tool for our mental health.

Medications and neurotransmitters

The medications most commonly prescribed for *depression* are selective serotonin reuptake inhibitors (SSRIs: Prozac, Paxil,

Zoloft, Celexa, Lexapro, etc.) and serotonin-norepinephrine reuptake inhibitors (SNRIs: Effexor, Cymbalta, Pristiq, etc.). These target and raise levels of the neurotransmitters serotonin and norepinephrine to improve mood and increase energy and alertness. The medications most commonly prescribed for general *anxiety* disorder are the Benzodiazepines (Xanax, Ativan, Valium, Librium, Klonipin, etc.), which are strong activators of GABA, the major inhibitory neurotransmitter that increases calmness and relaxation.

GABA

Gamma-aminobutyric acid (GABA) is an amino acid known as the primary inhibitory neurotransmitter in the mature brain after age 25. It is excitatory in the younger brain, which may be the reason children can have a "paradoxical response" to relaxing oils like lavender. Perhaps this reaction is the oils stimulating, not inhibiting, the GABA system in the younger brain.

GABA, by inhibiting certain nerve signals in the brain, calms your nervous system down to help reduce fear, anxiety and stress. Without the right level of GABA in the body, conditions such as anxiety disorders may become worse. Problems with GABA signaling seem to play a role in disorders that affect mental health and the nervous system.

Medications to regulate GABA signaling, such as benzodiazepines for anxiety and barbiturates for sedation, are effective; however, they carry the risk of abuse and physical addiction, and combined with other substances, supplements or alcohol can cause respiratory depression or, in the worst-case scenario, death.

Serotonin

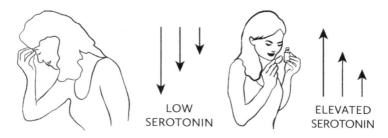

LOW
SEROTONIN

ELEVATED
SEROTONIN

Perhaps the best-known antidepressant neurotransmitter is serotonin; its main function is keeping our moods balanced, as well as being responsible for feelings of happiness and wellbeing. The majority of common antidepressants increase serotonin.

When levels of the stress hormone cortisol are decreased, serotonin levels increase, making you feel better. Aromatherapy inhalation decreases cortisol levels. Lavender has been the essential oil most studied, and is readily available, so is a good place to start the journey.

The body needs serotonin, but too much or too little can lead to health issues. For example, too little serotonin can lead to depression and too much can lead to a condition known as "serotonin syndrome," caused by too much antidepressant medication, combining medications for different conditions, or medication and herbal combinations all raising the serotonin levels. An example is a person taking an SSRI antidepressant such as Prozac and adding the herbal St John's Wort thinking that "natural is safe," when both increase levels of serotonin. The symptoms can vary in severity from agitation, confusion, insomnia, increased blood pressure and muscle rigidity to irregular heart rate and seizures. If this should happen, contact the physician or pharmacist or, if more serious, the

Emergency Room, as it can be life-threatening. The good news is that decreasing select medications with professional advice normally decreases symptoms.

Norepinephrine

Norepinephrine is a neurotransmitter and hormone that helps with alertness and energy, mood, memory, sleep-wake cycles and the "fight and flight" response.

Dopamine-D adrenergic system

Dopamine is the "feel-good" reward system hormone. With balanced dopamine levels, you have a sense of pleasure and this gives you the motivation and energy to accomplish tasks. Low levels are associated with attention deficit hyperactivity disorder (ADHD) and Parkinson's disease. High levels are associated with bipolar mania. Schizophrenia is associated with both too-high and too-low levels.

Cognitive effects have been improved with rosemary, clary sage and roman chamomile essential oils activating the dopamine-D adrenergic system (DA) (Wang and Heinbockel 2018).

Hypothalamic-Pituitary Axis

The hypothalamic-pituitary axis (HPA) "stress response system's" main function is the body's response to stress. As you experience stress, your adrenal glands make the hormone cortisol and release it into your bloodstream. Cortisol is known as the "stress hormone"; it triggers our fight and flight response, which increases pulse, blood pressure and feelings of anxiety, fear and, in some, panic. Women experience more intense menstrual issues, PMS and menopausal symptoms with increased stress. Aromatherapy is well known for its calming, stress-reducing properties, via the HPA, by reducing cortisol levels. When you inhale essential oils you're activating the pituitary gland which, through a cascade of responses, can improve hormonal and neurotransmitter levels, making you feel less anxious, irritable and improve your mood. Multiple studies (Atsumi and Tonosaki 2007; Heydari *et al.* 2018a; Pasyar, Rambod and Araghi 2020) indicate that inhalations of calming essential oils, such as lavender, rose, bergamot, grapefruit and more, affect the HPA, reducing elevated cortisol levels and increasing calming neurotransmitters.

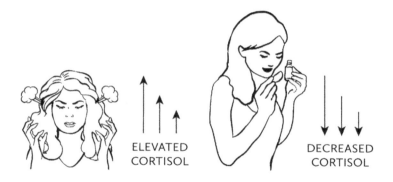

ELEVATED CORTISOL

DECREASED CORTISOL

Lizarraga-Valderrama's (2021) review of multiple animal and human essential oil (EO) studies indicated that inhalations of sweet orange, rose and lavender EOs reduced cortisol through the HPA, producing a sedative effect. Frankincense, ylang-ylang, bergamot, neroli, sweet orange, geranium and rose EOs can affect the HPA by decreasing cortisol levels, decreasing heart rate and blood pressure and calming anxiety. Aromatherapy, as a complementary therapy, offers a safe, pleasant and effective tool for mental health self-care and a supportive therapy for daily issues of depression, anxiety, focus, and cognitive and dementia conditions.

With chronic stress and persistent elevated cortisol via HPA, serotonin and dopamine levels are decreased, leading to anxiety disorders or depression. Ylang-ylang and rose EOs decrease cortisol levels, increasing serotonin levels and thus decreasing anxiety.

The concept of holistic medicine is viewing the person as a whole, interconnected living being and throughout this book there are multiple studies and relevant clinical experience unraveling the myriad of processes within a woman that contribute to her mental health and wellbeing. As a young nurse, I often heard references to patients at shift change reports which were not their names, but "the hysterectomy in room 202" "ovarian cancer in 204" "mastectomy in 206"—pieces and parts, not a whole thinking, feeling, functioning person. This reductionist language affects the collective female psyche. Is a woman just her reproductive organs? As a surgical nurse at a large medical center in charge of gynecology surgery for five years, the most common surgeries I saw were total hysterectomies (the removal of the uterus, ovaries and fallopian tubes). The rationale was that because there was an extremely low risk of the patient having ovarian cancer in the future which could require future surgery, it was better to, "Just take it all out now." This seemed strange to me as the majority of the women had suffered from uterine fibroids, heavy menstrual bleeding and pain, but rarely cancer, and ovarian cancer was not statistically that common. Later in my career, I encountered a number of women aged 40–55 who fell into deep depressions months after total hysterectomies. Most did not have previous histories of depression and were unaware and uninformed that this was a risk to this surgery. Had they been, they might not have consented to complete removal of their ovaries, as that removed their major source of estrogen. When hormonal levels fall, a cascade of events occur with other hormonal and neurotransmitter levels responding, leading to various physical and psychological effects. Often women were then prescribed synthetic hormones with accompanying risks, and pre-menopausal women were thrust into early menopause with hot flashes, foggy brains, decreased libido and unpleasant vaginal changes. Most of the women I encountered wished they had fully understood the interconnections and response of their whole being to this surgery and would've happily risked a potential, albeit unlikely, future surgery to have maintained their mental and physical health. Knowledge and education are so important, and a trusted relationship with the medical provider is invaluable; do your research and ask questions before a decision is made.

In the scenarios described above, aromatherapy is helpful to boost a sense of lost femininity and uplift feelings of depression. Use oils such as rose, lavender and jasmine by inhalation or a blend of two or three in a lotion which can be applied to the body. A spray with lavender and 1–2 drops of peppermint helps with hot flashes and can calm and uplift emotions. For a sense of overall hormonal balance and to decrease anger and irritability, a blend of ylang-ylang, geranium and clary sage by inhalation or diluted in lotion and applied to wrists, ankles and lower abdomen twice daily in practice provide comfort and balance.

Essential oils and neurotransmitters review summary

Recent human and animal studies highlighted in Wang and Heinbockel (2018) indicate that many essential oils used for anxiety have been shown to affect the functioning of the GABAergic system. Wang and Heinbockel (2018) focus on essential oils as an emerging promising source for modulation of the GABA system and their anxiolytic properties.

In addition to the GABAergic system, other neurotransmitter systems such as the serotonergic system have been shown to exert anxiolytic effects when activated by essential oils such as lavender (*lavandula angustifolia*) (Chioca *et al.* 2013).

Fung *et al.* (2021) noted that although most essential oils can interact with a range of neurotransmitter pathways (e.g., GABA, serotonin, noradrenergic, dopamine, etc.). the effect mainly depends on the effectiveness of their active components. The main method for human studies is by inhalation, and a summary of human studies is shown in the following table.

Human studies of clinical effects of common essential oil inhalations on anxiety and/or depression (based on Fung et al. 2021)

Essential oil	Anti-anxiety	Antidepressant	Clinical EO studies—Anxiety	Clinical EO studies—Depression
Lavender *Lavandula angustifolia*	X	X	Burnett *et al.* 2004, Lehrner *et al.* 2005, Fayazi *et al.* 2011, Senturk and Tekinsoy Kartin 2018, Karan 2019, Ebrahimi *et al.* 2021	Ebrahimi *et al.* 2021
Sweet orange *Citrus sinensis*	X	X	Lehrer *et al.* 2005, Goes *et al.* 2012	
Yuzu *Citrus junos*	X	X	Matsumoto *et al.* 2014	Matsumoto *et al.* 2014
Bergamot *Citrus bergamia*	X	X	Watanabe *et al.* 2015	
Chamomile	X	X	McKay and Blumberg 2006, Ebrahimi *et al.* 2021	McKay and Blumberg 2006 Ebrahimi *et al.* 2021

Rosemary *Salvia rosmarinus*	X		Burnett *et al.* 2004	
Lavender and rose *Lavandula angustifolia and rosa damescena*	X	X	Conrad and Adams 2012	Conrad and Adams 2012
Lavender, ylang-ylang and neroli *Lavandula angustifolia, cananga odorata and citrus aurantium*	X			Song and Lee (2018)

In summary, the most-prescribed pharmaceuticals for the treatment of anxiety and depression affect various neurotransmitter pathways to calm anxiety, improve mood and increase energy. Recent clinical studies of essential oils indicate that many essential oils affect the same neurotransmitter pathways and thus shine a light on their potential as tools to be used alone in milder conditions or alongside medications in more serious conditions; they offer valuable tools in the treatment of mental health conditions, most notably anxiety and depression.

CHAPTER 11

Clinical Case Studies

In over 20 years of my clinical aromatherapy nursing practice, there are numerous cases to highlight with the focus of emotional health treatment.

Disclaimer

The author wishes to express the importance of comprehensive mental healthcare and is not making any aromatherapy claims for cures or replacements for professional medical and psychological treatments. Aromatherapy is considered a complementary, not alternative therapy.

Nurses and midwives qualified in evidence-based aromatherapy conducted the case studies in clinical settings. In mental health, for the safety of our clients, it's important to understand professional boundaries and practice as a team to minimize risks and ensure the best outcomes. If a person expresses suicidal or homicidal thoughts or tendencies, connect them immediately with a mental health crisis team.

Cancer group therapy—active cancer therapy patients

A multicultural underserved breast cancer support group of 15 women in active treatment met weekly from 1 to 3 p.m. in a medical center conference room. None of them had previously been introduced to aromatherapy. As fatigue and nausea are frequent side-effects of cancer treatments, I diffused a blend of peppermint, rosemary and sweet orange for 15 minutes prior to and at the beginning of the group. There were no objections to the smell over two years, and no one became ill or fell asleep during the group.

At the end of each group, I offered either lavender or mandarin on a tissue or perfume strip for deep breathing and a guided imagery exercise. Several months into this practice, several shared that they took the scented tissue home with them and if anxious during the week smelt it and felt calmer.

Individual postpartum depression/thought disorder: "This blend is my crack"

An esteemed pharmaceutical scientist who was a participant in our postpartum depression study inhaled and applied lavender and rose in jojoba oil from the study (Conrad and Adams 2012) to her wrists as needed for several years postpartum to stay calm and less fearful. She would find me wherever I practiced to get her aroma blend, which seemed to be a necessary aspect of her comfort and recovery. Scent memories of comfort in troubled times can be supportive long term.

Bipolar hypomanic 51-year-old menopausal woman

A 51-year-old woman with a long history of noncompliant bipolar illness with frequent bouts of mania scheduled a massage in a clinic where I was a nurse aromatherapist consultant. She was irritable and insulting upon arrival and the staff were uncomfortable dealing with her. She was familiar to me as a past inpatient psychiatric patient and I was comfortable with her, though she didn't remember me. I offered her various scent strips to inhale. Negative and derogatory comments continued with each individual scent until she tried a menopausal blend of geranium, clary sage and ylang-ylang, which she kept inhaling. It significantly calmed her agitation and a somewhat pleasant demeaner emerged. She stated that she felt better and liked the scent. Her hormonal imbalance appeared to exacerbate her bipolar illness, and simple inhalations of the select oils calmed her, providing her with another option for rough patches on her long journey with bipolar illness. She left the appointment much calmer, with a bottle of the aromatherapy blend and instructions for use, as well as encouragement to contact her physician for follow-up mental health care .

Staff grief over death of beloved physician

Rose and frankincense on separate tissues passed amongst a group of grieving nurses in a church pew at the funeral of a much loved female OB/GYN physician eased sadness and comforted grief.

Panic attacks in young adult female

A professional 30-year-old female struggled periodically with anxiety and, at times, panic attacks. In addition to medication for anxious depression, a blend of equal amounts of neroli and frankincense in a personal inhaler reduced her anxiety from 7 to 3 on a Likert scale after just a few deep inhalations, and she kept it with her at work to help with her anxiety. If she was suffering from PMS, inhalations of a blend of clary sage, geranium, ylang-ylang and/or rose eased her irritability and calmed her.

Postpartum blues/depression in woman from Peru

A recent postpartum woman in Indiana without birth complications was, much to her husband's dismay, extremely sad to be far from her family in Peru. A cotton pad with jasmine 2 percent inhalation immediately brightened her mood as it reminded her of her mother's jasmine-filled garden in Peru; in her culture a mother would be nearby when her daughter gave birth. Her husband, astounded at her positive, rapid response and improved mood, requested a never-ending supply of the blend.

Woman with serotonin syndrome

A 55-year-old woman with a history of depression and grief had been diagnosed with serotonin syndrome, a very uncomfortable condition that occurs when high levels of the chemical serotonin accumulate in the body from specific antidepressants or combinations of medications. Serotonin is a chemical your body produces that's needed for your nerve cells and brain to function. But too much serotonin causes symptoms that can range from mild (shivering and diarrhea) to severe (muscle rigidity, fever and seizures). Severe serotonin syndrome can be fatal if not treated. After one month she hadn't had any relief with conventional medications for this condition. She was "jumping out of her skin," anxious and miserable.

She tried inhalation of frankincense (*boswellia carterii*), four drops on a cotton pad for four to five minutes. Her immediate response was "This is the most relief I've had from anything, it finally broke the cycle!" I sent her home with a bottle of frankincense and Bach flower Rescue Remedy to use four times a day and as needed. Two weeks later she returned and was doing very well, and had reduced her need to once a day and as needed.

Hidden alcoholic menopausal woman

A 55-year-old nurse and spouse of a physician who was curious about aromatherapy scheduled an appointment for mild menopausal symptoms. The session began with inhalation of a few essential oils, a bit like perfume sampling. She was chatting, deeply inhaled geranium oil, became emotional, started crying and blurted out, "I am an alcoholic." She stated that she hadn't planned to share this information, but once extremely relaxed by the aromatherapy could not keep it to herself. As a psychiatric nurse, I found this rather dramatic, a very rapid "peeling of the onion" compared to previous patients holding back their secrets as long as possible. She found the experience cathartic, and continued to use oils regularly for stress, anxiety and menopause as she started the journey towards treatment for her alcoholism. Many fears and insecurities surfaced in the following years, and she often made contact to request aromatherapy, mostly successfully, to ease her uncomfortable feelings while maintaining sobriety. At last contact, she was 10 years sober. This client taught me what a valuable therapeutic tool aromatherapy can be to open hidden passageways to the deepest secrets, and equally the need as a therapist to be prepared for an expedited process!

Divorce effects on spouse and pre-teen children

A 40-year-old, recently divorced, devout Catholic colleague with two preteen children contacted me for blends to give her strength and help her children sleep and cope with their new reality. They all were familiar with aromatherapy and the children requested their own personal blends.

Grief for her marriage, guilt from her Catholic faith and mild depression inspired a blend of frankincense, bergamot and jasmine—all calming oils she enjoyed, with evidence-based therapeutic antidepressant properties. She inhaled her blend as needed for several months with positive results. The 10–12-year-old male and female children each had the same blend of roman chamomile, lavender and ylang-ylang (unbeknownst to them) for sleep, anger and anxiety, with their individual names on the labels. Their sleep improved; they felt special with their own blends and empowered to determine when it was needed for their self-care, which also helped their mother know when they were struggling.

Infertility client

A 34-year-old teacher with infertility issues preparing for her second and final IVF treatment sought aromatherapy for emotional support. The journey had been long and costly and she and her husband were both struggling with fear, anxiety and anticipatory grief for the loss of their dream to have children of their own. She confirmed that she was not pregnant and received a massage with rose and geranium oils diluted to 4 percent in lotion for relaxation, grief and endocrine balance. For an ongoing support program, she used the same blend for couples' massages and a bath blend, with a goal of two baths and two massages each weekly for the remaining two weeks prior to IVF. The IVF treatment was successful, she became pregnant and although it is not possible to give credit to the aromatherapy, they were in a much more relaxed state than previous attempts. Since that time, studies have gone deeper to demonstrate the effect various essential oil constituents have on the endocrine and neurological hormonal and neurotransmitter pathways. What is understood with any condition is that a body functions better in a non-stressed state and, by all accounts, the couple were both more relaxed with the help of aromatherapy.

Individual just diagnosed with cancer, pre-procedure

A 38-year-old woman just diagnosed with breast cancer returned to the clinic the following day for a needle biopsy. Fearful, anxious and shaking, she was sent to me to calm her before the procedure. With a calm voice, I encouraged her to close her eyes and take slow deep breaths while she received a five-minute hand massage with 2 percent lavender diluted in lotion. Remarkably calmer within ten minutes of meeting, she indicated she felt better, cared for and more relaxed, and was ready for the procedure.

Grief with sleeplessness after death of mother

A 35-year-old female, full-time pharmacist, wife and mother of two young children revered and was best friends with her mother, a long-term breast cancer survivor. Devastated when the cancer returned and took her mother's life within a few short months, she found her normally high-functioning self unable to cope with the grief, anger and sleeplessness at night. Under a physician's care, she was prescribed antidepressants and sleep medication and found her incredibly sharp mind in a constant fog. Rather dismissive about complementary therapies, she was reluctant to try aromatherapy. However, she stopped her sleep medication and used a diffuser on her bedside table with a customized blend of roman chamomile, ylang-ylang and lavender. The oils in the blend were chosen for their varied sedative therapeutic properties. After a week of greatly improved sleep, she shared the positive effects of using this blend in her diffuser. She continued this practice successfully at home for two years with intermittent travel and overnights without it. A person of a few words, her referrals of pharmacy clients, family and friends for emotional support with aromatherapy was affirming.

Cancer support group anxiety study

A multicultural medical center breast cancer support group of 12 women had been meeting weekly for six months. Curious if aromatherapy could ease anxiety and thus enhance deeper discussions about life and death, intimacies and fears associated with cancer, we started a six-week study. Allergies were checked, consents were obtained and each week a diffuser was turned on in the group room. The members and facilitator were unaware if anything was in the diffuser on any given week. There were two weeks without any oils, two weeks with mandarin and lavender, and two with lavender and frankincense. Amusingly, group members always believed they smelled oils even if there weren't any. Likert scales measured each member before and after group responses. The facilitator noticed changes in group dynamics and behaviors on weeks that coincided with oils being diffused. The weeks of lavender and mandarin were more cheerful, with increased sharing and laughter. The frankincense and lavender weeks were more labile and emotional with increased crying and flights of ideas, and were much more difficult to facilitate. The participants rated their anxiety as decreased and their ability to communicate improved on the days that coincided with essential oils being diffused, particularly the lavender and mandarin sessions.

As noted throughout the book, various essential oils can uplift depressed moods or quell anxiety and panic in most people, by stimulating or calming.

For example, always consider the potential intensifying effects of the menstrual cycle, PMS, menopause, pregnancy, postpartum and chose oils that have been effective during these times (see tables).

Otherwise, if a person is depressed, fatigued, lethargic, and low energy, oils that are sedative wouldn't be the best choice. Instead, try non-sedating oils, such as bergamot, geranium, sweet orange or rose, to lift the mood without sedation. However, if irritability or insomnia accompany the depression, more sedative oils such as lavender, chamomile or ylang-ylang are a better choice. In times of heightened anxiety or panic, add inhalations of neroli and/or frankincense.

CHAPTER 12

Tried and Tested Basic Blends for Emotional Support

Inhalation is the quickest, most effective and evidence-based method of aromatherapy to relieve anxiety, panic and depression. In hospitals or institutions it is often more practical to use a diffuser or room spray: indirect inhalation.

Blend the essential oils together first, then inhale as a blend or, if using a lotion, dilute the blend in the lotion to apply to the body: 2–3 drops per teaspoonful of lotion.

Below are a few blends with the number of drops that women have found helpful. Try them and see what works for you and those in your care!

- Lavender 4, lemon 1

- Frankincense 4, lemon 1

- Lavender 4, rose 1

- Lavender 6, jasmine 2

- Lavender 4, jasmine 2, rose 1

- Bergamot 3, ylang-ylang 1, grapefruit 1

- Frankincense 2, orange 3, geranium 1

- Neroli 2, petitgrain 2, sweet orange2

- Bergamot 5, frankincense 4, jasmine 2

- Geranium 3, rosemary 2, lemon 1

- Lavender 3, roman chamomile 2, ylang-ylang 1

- Geranium 3, clary sage 3, ylang-ylang 3, rose 1

- Mandarin 1, sweet orange 1, lemon 1, grapefruit 1

Pediatric Supplement for Moms

According to the American Academy of Pediatrics:

> The worsening crisis in child and adolescent mental health is inextricably tied to the stress brought on by COVID-19 and the ongoing struggle for racial justice and represents an acceleration of trends observed prior to 2020. Rates of childhood mental health concerns and suicide rose steadily between 2010 and 2020 and by 2018 suicide was the second leading cause of death for youth ages 10–24. The pandemic has intensified this crisis: across the country we have witnessed dramatic increases in Emergency Department visits for all mental health emergencies including suspected suicide attempts.
>
> The pandemic has struck at the safety and stability of families, communities and societies. More than 140,000 children in the United States lost a primary and/or secondary caregiver, with youth of color disproportionately impacted. We are caring for young people with soaring rates of depression, anxiety, trauma, loneliness, and suicidality that will have lasting impacts on them, their families, and their communities. We must identify

strategies to meet these challenges through innovation and action, using state, local and national approaches to improve the access to and quality of care across the continuum of mental health promotion, prevention, and treatment. (American Academy of Pediatrics 2021)

Aromatherapy is effective, safe and well received by children and young adults with multiple stresses, anxiety, focus/attention, mild depression and grief. Along with professional psychological evaluation and treatment, creating a self-care aromatherapy remedy can be helpful. Younger children respond well to citrus, such as mandarin or sweet orange in a spritzer or diffuser, for both calming and uplifting. Preteens and teens can try the addition of bergamot, lavender and/or neroli for calming; rosemary and mint for focus; and ylang-ylang for issues with anger. Sweet orange is uplifting, pleasant and familiar as a scent related to a popular food so can ease the unpleasantness and fear of a clinical setting.

Pediatric aromatherapy for moms

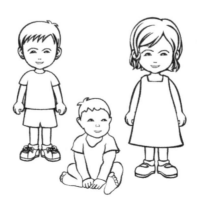

Safety

- Essential oils are very concentrated (e.g., 1 drop of peppermint essential oil = 28 tea bags).

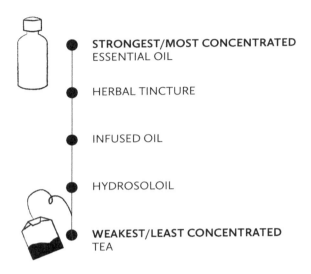

STRONGEST/MOST CONCENTRATED
ESSENTIAL OIL

HERBAL TINCTURE

INFUSED OIL

HYDROSOLOIL

WEAKEST/LEAST CONCENTRATED
TEA

- Only very small amounts should be used on young children.

- *External* use only (*never ingest*).

- *Always* dilute in lotion, aloe gel or carrier oil before applying to skin (avoid on suture lines or open wounds).

- *Avoid* essential oils before three months of age (for a normal-term infant).

- *Avoid* with asthma or allergies to essentials oil and/or related plants.

- *Avoid* peppermint and strong menthol essential oils

around infants and children under three years of age (potential for respiratory distress/arrest).

Methods

- Inhalation: Diluted drop/s on cotton pad, inhaler, diffuser or vaporizer.

- Skin application: Dilute in lotion, jojoba or grapeseed oil or aloe gel and apply directly to affected area or area of discomfort.

- Baths: Dilute 1–4 drops in whole milk, jojoba oil or Epsom salt and add to the filled tub just before entering. Soak for 10–20 minutes.

- Spritzer: Add 10–20 drops of essential oil to a 4 oz glass spray bottle, then fill to the neck with sterile or distilled water. Spray in room for calming emotions, focus and/ or for viral conditions.

For babies over three months of age and young children use gentle single essential oils such as:

- lavender

- roman chamomile

- mandarin

- rose otto.

Preferred safest amounts by the weight of the child for diluted essential oils added to a bath or one-time external diluted treatments (Price and Price 1996):

- 14–28 lbs   1 drop

- 28–56 lbs   2 drops

- 56–84 lbs   3 drops

- 84–112 lbs   4 drops

Avoid before 3 months of age.

If using for regular treatments over a period, use the following:

- Three months–one year   5 drops essential oil per 50 ml lotion

- One year and over   8 drops essential oil per 50 ml lotion

"A mother is only as happy as her saddest child."

Pediatric support

Basic conditions and treatment tips for children and moms:

- A bit like oxygen masks on planes, treat yourself first as suffering children increase our anxiety and irritability!

- Mothers can inhale any of the following on a cotton pad to calm yourself: lavender, rose, mandarin, geranium, ylang-ylang.

Colic

Roman chamomile alone or with mandarin

- Unscented white lotion.

- Dilute as per weight chart above and rub on lower back and clockwise on abdomen and bottom of feet.

Insomnia/sleep difficulties

Roman chamomile, lavender and/or mandarin

- Unscented white lotion.

- Bath before bed: 1–2 drops roman chamomile in jojoba or whole milk, pour into bath just before entering (every other night for 1 week, then 2–3 times the following week, then sleep should be improved).

- Skin application: Back, shoulder or arm bedtime massage with diluted roman chamomile, lavender and/or mandarin based on age/weight.

- Diluted drop of lavender, mandarin or both on cotton pad inside pillowcase or on stuffed animal (beware, mandarin will stain).

Try either skin application or drops or both every other night for one week, then 2–3 times the following week, then sleep should be improved; then only use as needed.

Anxiety/stress

Lavender, mandarin, roman chamomile, ylang-ylang (anger), frankincense (panic)

- Inhalation: 1–2 drops on cotton pad and inhale as needed.

- Room diffuser: Add 2–6 drops undiluted essential oils to diffuser.

- Room spritzer: 4–10 drops per 2–4 oz glass spray bottle, fill with distilled or sterile water; shake before use. Avoid eyes; spray around room, person or on sheets for rest.

- Bath: as for insomnia/sleep difficulties.

- Skin application/massage: as for insomnia/sleep difficulties.

Mild depression

Lavender, sweet orange, mandarin, lemon, bergamot

- Methods same as with anxiety and stress.

Grief

Lavender, frankincense, rose, lemon

- Inhalations, room diffusers and spritzers are helpful for children after divorce or deaths of friends, family or pets (lemon helps soften the frankincense or rose, which are both helpful for grief).

+ Sometimes letting the child smell a variety of oils and choose their own single oil or blend is nice.

ADD/ADHD/focus

Rosemary, peppermint, lemon (focus)

Lavender, mandarin, roman chamomile, sweet marjoram (calming)

+ Inhalation: 1–2 drops on cotton pad or personal inhaler.

+ Room diffuser: 2–6 drops and diffuse in study area.

+ Spritzer: 4–10 drops per 2–4 oz glass spray bottle, fill with distilled or sterile water; shake before use. Avoid eyes; spray around room or person as needed for focus and study.

Aches/pain/cramps

Lavender, sweet marjoram, roman chamomile, rosemary

+ Inhalation: 1–2 drops on a cotton pad for calming and decreased pain perception.

+ Skin application: Dilute in unscented white lotion or aloe gel and generously apply directly to area of discomfort as needed.

+ *Lavender:* Analgesic.

+ *Sweet marjoram:* Good for muscle/overuse pain.

- *Roman chamomile:* Good for muscle, abdominal/ "tummy" and young teen menstrual cramps.

Recommended pediatric clinical aromatherapy essential oil list

- Lavender
- Mandarin
- Lemon
- Sweet orange
- Rose
- Bergamot
- Roman chamomile
- Sweet marjoram
- Frankincense
- Rosemary
- Mint (only with children over 3 years of age)

Resources

The author does not have an affiliation with a particular essential oil company and, after 23 years of international clinical practice, shares the resources she has used and would recommend for personal and clinical practice.

Bottles and inhalers

- SKS Bottle & Packaging Inc. www.sks-bottle.com

- Specialty Bottle www.specialtybottle.com

Essential oils used by nurses in clinical aromatherapy programs

- Arlys Naturals www.arlysnaturals.com

- Absolute Aromas www.absolute-aromas.com

- Nature's Gift www.naturesgift.com

- Aromatics International www.aromatics.com

- Florihana www.florihana.com

- Oshadhi www.oshadhi.com (available in shops)

Nursing, mental health and aromatherapy organizations

- American Psychiatric Nurses Association (APNA) www.apna.org

- Association of Women's Health and Neonatal Nurses (AWHONN) www.awhonn.org

- Postpartum Support International (PSI) www.postpartum.net

- International Clinical Aromatherapy Network (ICAN) www.clinicalaromatherapynetwork.com

- National Institute of Mental Health (NIMH) www.nimh.nih.gov

- Alliance of International Aromatherapists (AIA) www.alliance-aromatherapists.org

- Canadian Federation of Aromatherapists (CFA) www.cfacanada.com

- National Association for Holistic Aromatherapy (NAHA) www.naha.org

- International Federation of Professional Aromatherapists (IFPA) www.ifparoma.org

Clinical aromatherapy published studies

Readers can filter all the articles to find those on subjects they are interested in.

- Pubmed www.ncbi.nlm.nih.gov/pubmed

- Researchgate www.researchgate.net

- Cochrane database www.cochranelibrary.com

Author's Note

As a nurse and then as an aromatherapist, the thread of mental and emotional health has woven through virtually every clinical encounter and treatment I've delivered for more than 35 years. As a woman, mother, wife, daughter and friend, I know the layers of our identities, experiences, secrets, traumas, successes, dreams and, most importantly, connections to each other create a stunningly beautiful tapestry.

Halfway through writing this guidebook I injured my shoulder, had extensive surgery and was unable to write for three months. The analogy of continuing with "one arm in a sling" aligned with women functioning as well as possible without all their resources. This seemed quite fitting for a book about women's mental health so, with the support and encouragement of my editor Carole, I chose to continue to the best of my ability. I sincerely hope you are positively informed and comforted in some measure by the content.

Aromatherapy has been an invaluable, pleasant and effective healthcare tool for thousands of women experiencing emotional, hormonal and physical discomforts. It is *nearly* impossible for most women to experience complete joy and contentment when one of their children is suffering, so often, sorting the child's (or partner, spouse, parent, sister or friend's) issues first demanded my attention prior to the woman being receptive to her own self-care. Most women are nurturers and experience wide ranges of emotions on any given day. All of this is normal; however, longer-term caregiving, losses, traumas, and lack of support and equal resources, coupled with hormonal shifts, take their toll on women's mental health. The range of females I've successfully treated in my years as a nurse aromatherapist include teens, college athletes, pregnant, laboring and postpartum women and cancer patients, as well as those experiencing depression, anxiety, panic, menopause, hospice and end of life. Many times, a brief encounter with select inhalation of oils relieved nausea, fear, anxiety and sleep, and at other times, aromatherapy provided a bridge of compassion for crisis survival until therapy or hospitalization was accomplished. Women are very strong and forming a bond of support with each other guides us through most of life's challenges. Aromatherapy is a valuable and pleasant tool in the large kit of mental health care. It's a bit like sharing a bouquet with each other, flower by flower until we choose a favorite, put it in a vase, take a breath and enjoy the simple bliss of Mother Nature's aromatic gifts to us!

Aromatic blessings to you and those in your care!

Pam

References

Abdelhakim, A. *et al.* (2020) The effect of inhalation aromatherapy in patients undergoing cardiac surgery: A systematic review and meta-analysis of randomized controlled trials. *Complementary Therapies in Medicine.*

Altemus, M., Saravaya, N. and Epperson, N. (2014) Sex differences in anxiety and depression clinical perspectives. *Frontiers in Neuroendocrinoloy 35, 3, 320–330.*

Amadeo, S. *et al.* (2020) Supportive effect of body contact care with ylang ylang aromatherapy and mobile intervention team for suicide prevention: A pilot study. *Journal of International Medical Research.*

American Academy of Pediatrics (2021) AAP-AACAP-CHA Declaration of a National Emergency in Child and Adolescent Mental Health. Accessed on 12/16/22 at www.aap.org/en/advocacy/child-and-adolescent-healthy-mental-development/aap-aacap-cha-declaration-of-a-national-emergency-in-child-and-adolescent-mental-health.

Anxiety and Depression Association of America (ADAA) (2022) Generalized Anxiety Disorder (GAD). Accessed on 01/23/23 at https://adaa.org/understanding-anxiety/generalized-anxiety-disorder-gad.

Anxiety and Depression Association of America (ADAA) (2023) PMS and PPD. Accessed on 03/31/23 at https://adaa.org/find-help-for/women/pms-pmdd.

Atsumi, T. and Tonosaki, K. (2007) Smelling lavender and rosemary increases free radical scavenging activity and decreases cortisol level in saliva. *Psychiatry Research.*

Asazawa, K. *et al.* (2017) The effect of aromatherapy treatment on fatigue and relaxation for mothers during the early puerperal period in Japan: A pilot study. *International Journal of Community Based Nursing and Midwifery 5*, 4, 365–375.

Babakhanian, M. *et al.* (2018) Effect of aromatherapy on the treatment of psychological symptoms in postmenopausal and elderly women: A systematic review and meta-analysis. *Journal of Menopausal Medicine.*

Ballard, C.G. *et al.* (2002) Aromatherapy as a safe and effective treatment for the management of agitation in severe dementia: The results of a double-blind, placebo-controlled trial with Melissa. *Journal of Clinical Psychiatry*, July.

Bastard, J. and Tiran, D. (2005) Aromatherapy and massage for antenatal anxiety: Its effect on the fetus. *Complementary Therapies in Clinical Practice 12*, 1, 48–54.

Beck, A. *et al.* (1988) An inventory for measuring clinical anxiety: Psychometric properties. *Journal of Consulting and Clinical Psychology.*

Bogdan, M.S. *et al.* (2021) Olfactory perception and different decongestive response of the nasal mucosa during menstrual cycle. *American Journal of Rhinology & Allergy*, January 26.

Burnett, K. *et al.* (2004) Scent and mood state following an anxiety-provoking task. *Psychological Reports.*

Burns, E.E. *et al.* (2000) An investigation into the use of aromatherapy in intrapartum midwifery practice. *Journal of Alternative and Complementary Medicine.*

Burns, E.E. *et al.* (2007) Aromatherapy in childbirth: A pilot randomised controlled trial. *BJOG: An International Journal of Obstetrics and Gynaecology.*

Centers for Disease Control and Prevention (2016/2017) National Intimate Partner and Sexual Violence Survey 2016/2017. Accessed on 01/02/23 at www.cdc.gov/violenceprevention/datasources/nisvs/summaryreports.html.

Centers for Disease Control and Prevention (2022a) About Mental Health. Accessed on 01/23/23 at www.cdc.gov/mentalhealth/learn/index.htm.

Centers for Disease Control and Prevention (2022b) Morbidity and Mortality Weekly Report (*MMWR*). Mental health, suicidality, and connectedness among high school students during the COVID-19 pandemic Adolescent behaviors and experiences survey, United

States, January–June 2021. Accessed on 01/23/23 at www.cdc.gov/mmwr/volumes/71/su/su7103a3.htm.

Centers for Disease Control and Prevention (2022c) Abortion Surveillance—Findings and Reports. Accessed on 03/31/23 at https://www.cdc.gov/reproductivehealth/data_stats/abortion.htm.

Centers for Disease Control and Prevention (2023) What is Infertility? Accessed on 03/31/23 at https://www.cdc.gov/reproductivehealth/features/what-is-infertility/index.html#common.

Chand, S. and Marwaha, R. (2022) *Anxiety*. Treasure Island, FL: StatPearls Publishing.

Chang, S. (2008) Effects of aroma hand massage on pain, state anxiety and depression in hospice patients with terminal cancer. *Taehan Kanho Hakhoe Chi 38*, 4, 493–502.

Chen, M.L. *et al.* (2022) The effect of bergamot essential oil aromatherapy on improving depressive mood and sleep quality in postpartum women: A randomized controlled trial. *Journal of Nursing Research.*

Chida, Y. and Steptoe, A. (2009) The association of anger and hostility with future coronary heart disease: A meta-analytic review of prospective evidence. *Journal of the American College of Cardiology 53*, 11, 936–946.

Cho, M. *et al.* (2103) Effects of aromatherapy on the anxiety, vital signs, and sleep quality of percutaneous coronary intervention patients in intensive care units. *Evidence Based Complementary Alternative Medicine.*

Chioca, L.R. *et al.* (2013) Anxiolytic-like effect of lavender essential oil inhalation in mice: Participation of serotonergic but not GABA/benzodiazepine neurotransmission. *Journal of Ethnopharmacology.*

Conrad, P. and Adams, C. (2012) The effects of clinical aromatherapy for anxiety and depression in the high risk postpartum woman—a pilot study. *Complementary Therapies in Clinical Practice.*

Costa, C. *et al.* (2011) The GABAergic system contributes to the anxiolytic-like effect of essential oil from Cymbopogon citratus (lemongrass). *Journal of Ethnopharmacology.*

Deng *et al.* (2022) Aromatherapy plus music therapy improve pain intensity and anxiety scores in patients with breast cancer during perioperative periods. *Clinical Breast Cancer 22*, 2, 115–120.

Department of Health and Human Services/Centers for Disease Control and Prevention (2021) Morbidity and Mortality Weekly Report (MMWR). June 18, vol. 70, no. 24.

Dugas, C. and Slane, V.H. (2022) *Miscarriage.* Treasure Island, FL: Stat-Pearls Publishing.

Ebrahimi, H. *et al.* (2021) The effects of Lavender and Chamomile essential oil inhalation aromatherapy on depression, anxiety and stress in older community-dwelling people: A randomized controlled trial. *Explore (NY).*

Es-haghee, S. *et al.* (2020) The effects of aromatherapy on premenstrual syndrome symptoms: A systematic review and meta-analysis of randomized clinical trials. *Evidence-Based Complementary and Alternative Medicine.* https://doi.org/10.1155/2020/6667078.

Fayazi, S., Babashahi, M. and Rezaei, M. (2011) The effect of inhalation aromatherapy on anxiety level of the patients in preoperative period. *Iranian Journal of Nursing and Midwifery Research.*

Fornaro, M. *et al.* (2019) The FDA "black box" warning on antidepressant suicide risk in young adults: More harm than benefits? *Frontiers in Psychiatry 10,* 294.

Fung, T. *et al.* (2021) Therapeutic effect and mechanisms of essential oils in mood disorders: Interaction between the nervous and respiratory systems. *International Journal of Molecular Science.*

Geethanjali, S. *et al.* (2020) Effect of clary sage oil as an aromatherapy on cardiac autonomic function among patients with premenstrual syndrome—a randomized controlled study. *Obesity Medicine.*

Goes, T. *et al.* (2012) Effect of sweet orange aroma on experimental anxiety in humans. *Journal of Alternative and Complementary Medicine.*

Gordon, B. (1979) *I'm Dancing as Fast as I Can.* New York: Bantam Books.

Graham, P.H. *et al.* (2003) Inhalation aromatherapy during radiotherapy: Results of a placebo-controlled double-blind randomized trial. *Journal of Clinical Oncology.*

Granger, R., Campbell, E. and Johnston, G. (2005) (+)- And (-)-borneol: Efficacious positive modulators of GABA action at human recombinant α1β2γ2L GABAA receptors. *Biochemical Pharmacology,* April.

Han, X. *et al.* (2017) Bergamot (Citrus bergamia) essential oil inhalation improves positive feelings in the waiting room of a mental health treatment center: A pilot study. *Phytotherapy Research.*

Her, J. and Cho, M.K. (2021) Effect of aromatherapy on sleep quality of adults and elderly people: A systematic literature review and meta-analysis. *Complementary Therapies in Medicine.*

Heydari, N. *et al.* (2018a) Evaluation of aromatherapy with essential oils of Rosa damascena for the management of premenstrual syndrome. *International Journal of Gynecology and Obstetrics.*

Heydari, N. *et al.* (2018b) Investigation of the effect of aromatherapy with Citrus aurantium blossom essential oil on premenstrual syndrome in university students: A clinical trial study. *Complementary Therapies in Clinical Practice.*

Heydari, N. *et al.* (2019) The effect of aromatherapy on mental, physical symptoms, and social functions of females with premenstrual syndrome: A randomized clinical trial. *Journal of Family Medicine and Primary Care.*

Ho, D. (2012) Antidepressants and the FDA's black-box warning: Determining a rational public policy in the absence of sufficient evidence. *AMA Journal of Ethics,* June.

Holm, L. and Fitzmaurice, L. (2008) Emergency department waiting room stress: Can music or aromatherapy improve anxiety scores? *Pediatric Emergency Care.*

Hu, P. *et al.* (2010) Aromatherapy for reducing colonoscopy related procedural anxiety and physiological parameters: A randomized controlled study. *Hepatogastroenterology.*

Hur, K. *et al.* (2018) Association of alterations in smell and taste with depression in older adults. *Laryngoscope Investigative Otolaryngology* 3, 2 94–99.

Imanishi, J. *et al.* (2009) Anxiolytic effect of aromatherapy massage in patients with breast cancer. *Evidence Based Complementary Alternative Medicine 6,* 1, 123–128.

Ipek, C. (2004) AROMATERAPI: Kokunun gücü.

Jones, I. (2020) Postpartum psychosis: an important clue to the etiology of mental illness. *World Psychiatry 19,* 3. 334–336.

Kang, H.-J. *et al.* (2019) How strong is the evidence for the anxiolytic efficacy of lavender? Systematic review and meta-analysis of randomized controlled trials. *Asian Nursing Research,* December.

Karan, N.B. (2019) Influence of lavender oil inhalation on vital signs and anxiety: A randomized clinical trial. *Physiology and Behavior.*

Kasper, S. *et al.* (2010). Silexan, an orally administered Lavandula oil preparation, is effective in the treatment of "subsyndromal" anxiety disorder: A randomized, double-blind, placebo controlled trial. *International Clinical Psychopharmacology 25,* 277–287.

Kasper, S. *et al.* (2014). Lavender oil preparation Silexan is effective in generalized anxiety disorder: A randomized, double-blind comparison to placebo and paroxetine. *International Journal of Neuropsychopharmacology 17,* 859–869.

Kianpour, M. *et al.* (2016) Effect of lavender scent inhalation on prevention of stress, anxiety and depression in the postpartum period. *Iranian Journal of Nursing and Midwifery Research.*

Kianpour, M. *et al.* (2018) The effects of inhalation aromatherapy with rose and lavender at week 38 and postpartum period on postpartum depression in high-risk women referred to selected health centers of Yazd, Iran in 2015. *Iranian Journal of Nursing and Midwifery Research.*

Kim, M. *et al.* (2021) Effects of lavender on anxiety, depression, and physiological parameters: Systematic review and meta-analysis. *Asian Nursing Research.*

Koo, B.S. *et al.* (2004) Inhibitory effects of the essential oil from SuHeXiang Wan on the central nervous system after inhalation. *Biological and Pharmaceutical Bulletin.*

Koohpayeh, S. *et al.* (2021) Effects of *Rosa damascena* (Damask rose) on menstruation-related pain, headache, fatigue, anxiety, and bloating: A systematic review and meta-analysis of randomized controlled trials. *Journal of Education and Health Promotion.*

Lehrner, J. *et al.* (2005) Ambient odors of orange and lavender reduce anxiety and improve mood in a dental office. *Physiology and Behavior 86,* 1–2, 92–95.

Lizarraga-Valderrama, L.R. (2021) Effects of essential oils on the central nervous system: Focus on mental health. *Phytotherapy Research.*

Lotfipur-Rafsanjani, S.M. *et al.* (2018) Effects of geranium aromatherapy massage on premenstrual syndrome: A clinical trial. *International Journal of Preventative Medicine.*

Lv, X.N. *et al.* (2013) Aromatherapy and the central nerve system (CNS): Therapeutic mechanism and its associated genes. *Current Drug Targets,* July.

Mannucci, C. *et al.* (2018) Clinical pharmacology of *Citrus aurantium* and *Citrus sinensis* for the treatment of anxiety. *Evidence Based Complementary Alternative Medicine.*

Marzouk, T., El-Nemer, A. and Baraka, H.N. (2013) The effect of aromatherapy abdominal massage on alleviating menstrual pain in nursing students: A prospective randomized cross-over study. *Evidence Based Complementary and Alternative Medicine.*

Matsumoto, T., Asakura, H. and Hayashi, T. (2013) Does lavender aromatherapy alleviate premenstrual emotional symptoms? A randomized crossover trial. *BioPsychoSocial Medicine.*

Matsumoto, T., Asakura, H. and Hayashi, T. (2014) Effects of olfactory stimulation from the fragrance of the Japanese citrus fruit yuzu (Citrus junos Sieb. ex Tanaka) on mood states and salivary chromogranin A as an endocrinologic stress marker. *Journal of Alternative and Complementary Medicine.*

Matsumoto, T., Kimura, T. and Hayashi, T. (2016) Aromatic effects of a Japanese citrus fruit—yuzu (Citrus junos Sieb. ex Tanaka)—on psycho emotional states and autonomic nervous system activity during the menstrual cycle: A single-blind randomized controlled crossover study. *BioPsychoSocial Medicine.*

Mattina, G.F., Van Lieshoust, R.J. and Steiner, M. (2019) Inflammation, depression and caridovascular disease in women: The role of the immune system across critical reproductive events. *Therapeutic Advances in Cardiovascular Disease 13*, 1–26.

McKay, D. and Blumberg, J. (2006) A review of the bioactivity and potential health benefits of chamomile tea (Matricaria recutita L.). *Phytotherapy Research.*

Mohebitabar, S. *et al.* (2017) Therapeutic efficacy of rose oil: A comprehensive review of clinical evidence. *Avicenna Journal of Phytomedicine.*

Moslemi, F. *et al.* (2019) *Citrus aurantium* aroma for anxiety in patients with acute coronary syndrome: A double-blind placebo-controlled trial. *Journal of Alternative and Complementary Medicine.*

Nair, R. *et al.* (2021) Characteristics and outcomes of early recurrent myocardial infarction after acute myocardial infarction. *Journal of the American Heart Association 10*, 16.

National Alliance on Mental Illness (NAMI) (2022) Mental Health by the Numbers. Accessed on 01/23/23 at www.nami.org/mhstats.

National Institute of Mental Health (NIMH) (2022a) Mental Illness. Accessed on 01/23/23 at www.nimh.nih.gov/health/statistics/mental-illness.

National Institute of Mental Health (NIMH) (2022b) Major Depression. Accessed on 01/23/23 at www.nimh.nih.gov/health/statistics/major-depression.

National Institute of Mental Health (NIMH) (2022c) Post-Traumatic Stress Disorder (PTSD). Accessed on 01/23/23 at www.nimh.nih.gov/health/statistics/ post-traumatic-stress-disorder-ptsd.

Ou, M.C. *et al.* (2012) Pain relief assessment by aromatic essential oil massage on outpatients with primary dysmenorrhea: A randomized, double-blind clinical trial. *Journal of Obstetrics and Gynaecology Research.*

Pasyar, N., Rambod, M. and Araghi, F. (2020) The effect of bergamot orange essence on anxiety, salivary cortisol, and alpha amylase in patients prior to laparoscopic cholecystectomy: A controlled trial study. *Complementary Therapies in Clinical Practice.*

Peters *et al.* (2021) Trends in recurrent coronary heart disease after myocardial infarction among US women and men between 2008 and 2017. *Circulation 143,* 7, 650–660.

Pew Research Center (2023) What the data says about abortion in the US. Accessed on 01/23/23 at www.pewresearch.org/fact-tank/2023/01/11/what-the-data-says-about-abortion-in-the-u-s-2.

Prasad, A. (2007) Apical ballooning syndrome: An important differential diagnosis of acute myocardial infarction. *Circulation 115,* 5, e56–e59.

Price, P. and Price, S. (1996) *Aromatherapy for Babies and Children.* London: Thorsons.

Rashidi, F. *et al.* (2013) The effects of aromatherapy on pain of labor in nulliparous women. *Journal of North Khorasan University of Medical Sciences.*

Sadeghi, H. *et al.* (2014) The effect of self-aromatherapy massage of the abdomen on the primary dysmenorrhea. *Journal of Obstetrics and Gynaecology,* 382–385.

Scandurra, C. *et al.* (2022) The effectiveness of neroli essential oil in relieving anxiety and perceived pain in women during labor: A randomized controlled trial. *Healthcare,* February.

Schmidt, K. *et al.* (2018) Anger and coronary artery disease in women submitted to coronary angiography: A 48-month follow-up. *Arquivos brasileiros de cardiologia 111,* 410–416.

Scuteri, D. *et al.* (2019) Neuropharmacology of the neuropsychiatric symptoms of dementia and role of pain: Essential oil of bergamot as a novel therapeutic approach. *International Journal of Molecular Science 20*, 13, 3327.

Seo, J.Y. *et al.* (2009) The effects of aromatherapy on stress and stress responses in adolescents. *Journal of Korean Academy of Nursing.*

Semahegn, A. *et al.* (2020) Psychotropic medication non-adherence and its associated factors among patients with major psychiatric disorders: A systematic review and meta-analysis. *Systemic Review.*

Senturk, A. and Tekinsoy Kartin, P. (2018) The effect of lavender oil application via inhalation pathway on hemodialysis patients' anxiety level and sleep quality. *Holistic Nursing Practice.*

Sheng, J. *et al.* (2021) The hypothalamic-pituitary-adrenal axis: Development, programming actions of hormones, and maternal-fetal interactions. *Frontiers in Behavioral Neuroscience*, 13 January.

Siddiqui, M.J. *et al.* (2014) Role of complementary and alternative medicine in geriatric care: A mini review. *Pharmacological Reviews.*

Smeijers, L. *et al.* (2017) Anxiety and anger immediately prior to myocardial infarction and long-term mortality: Characteristics of high-risk patients. *Journal of Psychosomatic Research 93*, 19–27.

Song, E.J. and Lee, M.Y. (2018) Effects of aromatherapy on stress responses, autonomic nervous system activity and blood pressure in the patients undergoing coronary angiography: A non-randomized controlled trial. *Journal of Korean Academy of Nursing.*

Spitzer, R. *et al.* (2006) A brief measure for assessing generalized anxiety disorder: The GAD-7. *Archives of Internal Medicine.*

Strawn, J.R. *et al.* (2018) Pharmacotherapy for generalized anxiety disorder in adults and pediatric patients: An evidence-based treatment review *19*, 10, 1057–1070.

Tasca, C. *et al.* (2012) Women and hysteria in the history of mental health. *Clinical Practice and Epidemiology in Mental Health 8*, 110–119.

Teicher, M.H., Glod, C. and Cole, J.O. (1990) Emergence of intense suicidal preoccupation during fluoxetine treatment. *American Journal of Psychiatry.*

Tola, Y.O., Ming Chow, K. and Liang, W. (2021) Effects of non-pharmacological interventions on preoperative anxiety and postoperative pain in patients undergoing breast cancer surgery. *Journal of Clinical Nursing 30*, 23–24.

Uehleke, B. *et al.* (2012) Phase II trial on the effects of Silexan in patients with neurasthenia, post-traumatic stress disorder or somatization disorder. *Phytomedicine 19*, 665–671.

US Office on Women's Health (2021) Mental health.

Uysal, M. *et al.* (2016) Investigating the effect of rose essential oil in patients with primary dysmenorrhea. *Complementary Therapies in Clinical Practice 24*, 45–49.

Uzunçakmak, T. and Alkaya, A. (2018) Effect of aromatherapy on coping with premenstrual syndrome: A randomized controlled trial. *Complementary Therapies in Medicine 36*, 63–67.

Van Brederode, J. *et al.* (2016) The terpenoids Myrtenol and Verbenol act on δ subunit-containing GABAA receptors and enhance tonic inhibition in dentate gyrus granule cells. *Neuroscience Letters.*

Xiao, S. *et al.* (2021) Effects of aromatherapy on agitation and aggression in cognitive impairment: A meta-analysis. *Journal of Clinical Nursing*, August.

Wang, Z.J. and Heinbockel, T. (2018) Essential oils and their constituents targeting the GABAergic system and sodium channels as treatment of neurological diseases. *Molecules 23*, 5, 1601.

Watanabe, E. *et al.* (2015) Effects of bergamot (Citrus bergamia (Risso) Wright & Arn.) essential oil aromatherapy on mood states, parasympathetic nervous system activity, and salivary cortisol levels in 41 healthy females. *Forsch Komplementmed 22*, 1, 43–49.

Watanabe, K., Umezu, K. and Kurahashi, T. (2002) Human olfactory contrast changes during the menstrual cycle. *Japanese Journal of Physiology*, 353–359.

WHO (2022) COVID-19 pandemic triggers 25% increase in prevalence of anxiety and depression worldwide. Accessed on 02/20/23 at www.who.int/news/item/02-03-2022-covid-19-pandemic-triggers-25-increase-in-prevalence-of-anxiety-and-depression-worldwide.

Wilkinson, S. *et al.* (2007) Effectiveness of aromatherapy massage in the management of anxiety and depression in patients with cancer: A multicenter randomized controlled trial. *Journal of Clinical Oncology*, February.

Woelk, H. and Schlafke, S. (2010) A multi-center, double-blind, randomised study of the lavender oil preparation Silexan in comparison to Lorazepam for generalized anxiety disorder. *Phytomedicine 17*, 94–99.

Young, J. MD (2015) Women and mental illness: Why are mental health issues more common among women? *Psychology Today*, April 22.

Made in the USA
Middletown, DE
18 August 2023

36619852R00086